MW00973175

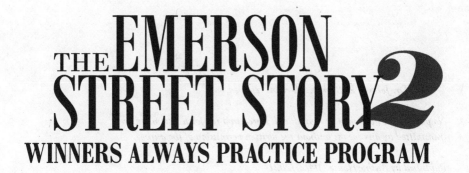

THE EMERSON STREET STORY 2
WINNERS ALWAYS PRACTICE PROGRAM

DR. JOHNNY E. BROWN

authorHOUSE

AuthorHouse™
1663 Liberty Drive
Bloomington, IN 47403
www.authorhouse.com
Phone: 833-262-8899

© 2021 Dr. Johnny E. Brown. All rights reserved.

No part of this book may be reproduced, stored in a retrieval system, or
transmitted by any means without the written permission of the author.

Published by AuthorHouse   04/27/2021

ISBN: 978-1-6655-2413-1 (sc)
ISBN: 978-1-6655-2414-8 (hc)
ISBN: 978-1-6655-2421-6 (e)

Library of Congress Control Number: 2021908502

Print information available on the last page.

Any people depicted in stock imagery provided by Getty Images are models,
and such images are being used for illustrative purposes only.
Certain stock imagery © Getty Images.

This book is printed on acid-free paper.

Because of the dynamic nature of the Internet, any web addresses or links contained in
this book may have changed since publication and may no longer be valid. The views
expressed in this work are solely those of the author and do not necessarily reflect the
views of the publisher, and the publisher hereby disclaims any responsibility for them.

Scripture quotations marked KJV are from the Holy Bible, King James Version
(Authorized Version). First published in 1611. Quoted from the KJV Classic
Reference Bible, Copyright © 1983 by The Zondervan Corporation.

Thank you very much to the editing team, led by Carolyn J. Brown and supported by Berlin Lee Brown for his insightful input. I am also extremely grateful to Reesha Johnette (Brown) Edwards for designing the book cover and Mary (Brown) Ruegg for designing the WAPP logo and graphics.

About the Book

This book is about the Winners Always Practice Program (WAPP), which is a set of tips on winning strategies for sports, games, and life. The information presented is beneficial to everyone, from childhood through adulthood on 21 components to consider which, when practiced, add joy and value to each day. Each component is aligned with ten biblical verses to tie the recommendations with a faith-based platform. The program was first introduced in the book, entitled: The Emerson Street Story: Race, Class, Quality of Life and Faith, published – August 2020. Following the recommendations for behaviors, practices, and actions dramatically increases the chances for success, happiness, and higher quality of life.

The author explains how practicing each of these categories and components each day positively affects relationships with others within and across race, class and otherwise. We can all succeed and get along with others by taking time to practice well established and accepted behaviors presented in the book.

Contents

Contents

Acknowledgements

I am delighted and honored to acknowledge the contributions of many colleagues, authors, family members, and friends who helped to guide my thoughts and influenced this project from start to finish. Thank you. Some have died and are no longer with us in a physical sense but continue to impact my views. I am grateful for the support of my colleagues: Faculties and staff of Lamar University and The University of Texas at Austin; Reverend Dr. John R. Adolph; Reverend Dr. Jack C. Gause; William C. Akins; Carolyn Bailey; Robert and Tanuya Worthy; Judge John Paul Stephens; Drs. Abbe Boring, Morcease Beasley, Ruben Olivarez, Stanton Lawrence, Walter Milton, Jr., Sharon Desmoulin-Kherat, Ameca Thomas, and Queinnise Miller. I am especially grateful for the assistance and support of my family: wife, Carolyn Jean (Reese) Brown; son, Berlin Lee Brown; daughters, Mary Katherine (Brown) Ruegg and Reesha Johnette (Brown) Edwards; son-in-law, Kyle Ruegg and parents, Steve and Robin Ruegg, and son-in-law, Desmond Edwards and parents; granddaughter, Abigail Sage Ruegg, and birth family members, including: mother, Mary Minnie (Bass) Brown, father, Lee Boyd Brown, Sr., sisters, Joyce Marie and Anita Lynne Brown, and brothers, Lee Boyd Brown, Jr., Willie Arthur and Anthony Wayne Brown and their spouses.

Writing this book has been truly a family affair and "labor of love". Thanks much to my wife, Carolyn, for the hours she devoted in book editing, especially for ensuring accuracy and appropriate language, clarity and writing style. And I am grateful for our son, Berlin Lee Brown, for his words of inspiration and consistent presence and philosophical utterances. Thanks also to our two daughters: Reesha Johnette (Brown) Edwards, the book cover designer; and Mary Katherine (Brown) Ruegg who was co-designer of the WAPP logo with the author. Thanks also to Gloria Hayes -- Darchase Designs – who produced the WAPP chart, in coordination with the author.

Introduction And Overview

Lift Ev'ry Voice and Sing

(Negro/Black National Anthem)

James Weldon Johnson
(1917)

Lift every voice and sing
Till earth and heaven ring,
Ring with the harmonies of Liberty;
Let our rejoicing rise
High as the listening skies,
Let it resound loud as the rolling sea.
Sing a song full of the faith that the dark past has taught us,
Sing a song full of the hope that the present has brought us.
Facing the rising sun of our new day begun,
Let us march on till victory is won.

Stony the road we trod,
Bitter the chastening rod,
Felt in the days when hope unborn had died;
Yet with a steady beat,
Have not our weary feet
Come to the place for which our fathers sighed?

We have come over a way that with tears has been watered,
We have come, treading our path through the blood of the slaughtered,
Out from the gloomy past,
Till now we stand at last
Where the white gleam of our bright star is cast.

God of our weary years,
God of our silent tears,
Thou who hast brought us thus far on the way;
Thou who hast by Thy might
Led us into the light,
Keep us forever in the path, we pray.
Lest our feet stray from the places, our God, where we met Thee,
Lest, our hearts drunk with the wine of the world, we forget Thee;
Shadowed beneath Thy hand,
May we forever stand.
True to our God,
True to our native land.
Our native land.

See below three of thousands of examples of inspirational
musical renditions of Lift Every Voice and Sing.

Model 1- youtube video by Spelman University Glee Club Choir – February, 2019

Model 2- youtube video by Huston Tillotson University Choir – April, 2016

Model 3- youtube video by The Balm In Gilead, Inc. – February, 2009

Each day is a new day and can bring fresh opportunities, hopes and dreams, while a person is standing tall for doing things in the right way and for the right reasons. Some of those hopes and dreams inevitably and coincidentally come true, and others come true only when a person devotes the time and attention to make it so. One such universal dream is the one on high quality of life, which everyone desires to experience. It is refreshing to dream and enjoy poems and songs that energize us toward rejoicing and imagining the world becoming a better place to live. This book presents ideas which are beneficial for everyone, from childhood through adulthood, regarding 21 behavioral components which, when practiced, add joy and value to each day: Winners Always Practice Program (WAPP). The road to travel for realizing the dream of more joy, less gloom and high quality of life is the adoption of the WAPP mentality. The program was first introduced in the book: The Emerson Street Story: Race, Class, Quality of Life and Faith, published – August 2020. There is no guessing about this, or assumptions being posited; rather, just a review of recommendations for behaviors, practices, and actions which lead to success, happiness, and high quality of life. Each category is aligned with ten biblical verses, and "faith" is intertwined throughout the program as a means for demonstrating relevance and significance.

The author deliberately limited the explanations to brief and common terms per category, while noting that all categories are important and that it makes a tremendous difference to "connect the dots" within and across each category. That is, no category is a "throw away" or insignificant area of importance -- practicing each component everyday enables a person to better enjoy life and happiness.

How do moments or memories fit into the picture? Moments in the context of this book refer to those special instances that are so profound they are etched into the mind and become memories, some positive and enlightening and others not so positive. Such memories -- positive and negative or frightening -- can often last a lifetime and influence a person's thoughts and actions. The more a person focuses on the positive experiences and moments, the more that person's outlook on life is predictably positive. The difference between success and failure is often controlled and determined by the way a person thinks and looks at the circumstances. The idea of thinking you can succeed is a giant step in the right direction toward the victory!

The following is a list of ten categories of the memorable moments in the life of the author that influenced the ideas and programmatic features shared in the WAPP.

- Participating in high school and college as an athlete -- basketball player -- representing the school and enjoying the public announcements of the author being named as the first college scholarship athlete of color.
- Education experiences growing up in Austin, Texas including elementary, junior high, and high school in segregated environments where school facilities in East Austin were inequitable compared with facilities in other parts of the city, and no new books were ever provided. Yet, employees and parents worked hard to inspire and encourage children to do the best work in learning and becoming educated.
- Learning how to drive and purchase of first car and each car afterwards and the purchase of the author's first house, followed by purchases of other houses.
- Graduation from college for each degree earned: B.S. in Education; M. Ed., and Ph. D.
- The joy and exhilarating feeling of being selected for the first teaching – coaching job and each job that followed as an educator.
- Wedding day in Paris, Texas and marriage to wife, Carolyn Jean (Reese) Brown and weddings of the author's two daughters.
- Birth of the author's son and two daughters.
- Notifications of when the author's children were selected for their colleges of choice and when they were offered their first professional employment opportunities.
- Family reunions and family gatherings at special times of the year, such as Christmas and Thanksgiving.
- Deaths and funerals of family members.

Definition of words commonly referred to in the book:

- Dream - a series of thoughts, images, or emotions occurring during sleep . . . a strongly desired goal or purpose.
- Memories - the power or process of reproducing or recalling what has been learned and retained . . . a particular act of recall or recollection.
- Moments - a minute portion or point of time . . . a comparatively brief period . . . a time of excellence or conspicuousness.

(Merriam-Webster, inc. – 2021)

Invictus

By William Ernest Henley
(1875)

Out of the night that covers me,
Black as the pit from pole to pole,
I thank whatever gods may be
For my unconquerable soul.

In the fell clutch of circumstance
I have not winced nor cried aloud.
Under the bludgeonings of chance
My head is bloody, but unbowed.

Beyond this place of wrath and tears
Looms but the Horror of the shade,
And yet the menace of the years
Finds and shall find me unafraid.

It matters not how strait the gate,
How charged with punishments the scroll,
I am the master of my fate,
I am the captain of my soul.

BIBLICAL REFERENCE ON FAITH

Now faith is the substance of things hoped for, the evidence of things not seen. For by it the elders obtained a good report. Through faith we understand that the worlds were framed by the word of God, so that things which are seen were not made of things which do appear. (Hebrews 11: 1-3)

Excerpts from: *The Emerson Street Story: Race, Class, Quality of Life and Faith.*

"*While growing up as a child I had visions of a world where equality meant equality for all, within and across all aspects of life, especially, in the United States of America. I wondered then, and I continue to question, the reasoning behind people being treated a certain way based upon class -- group classification or sorting according to commonly held beliefs on wealth, characteristics, historical understandings -- and race. I thought often about what role I could play to influence society toward such a reality of equality so that all concerned would enjoy a higher quality of life and happiness. My childhood experience was mostly one of joy and happiness and strength, undergirded by love of family, friends and Christianity. It was also a time of disappointment and regrets for how much we were, and continue to be, affected and driven by considerations of race, class, and social dynamics . . . We will all enjoy a higher quality of life when we focus more on the common good and less on considerations of race and class and selfish benefits. The appropriate and progressive way to look at diversity is to celebrate and appreciate it.*

The Brown family has come a long way since our experiences before and after we moved to the house located on Emerson Street. We were fortunate to always enjoy nice houses to live in -- Comal Street, Emerson Street and more recently, Basford Road. When we lived on Comal Street, we had three bedrooms, a den, a courtyard, and a fishpond, with fish in it, where neighbors and friends ... fished. The pond was encircled by bricks, giving it a very pleasing appearance. This structure was put in place in the 1940s, and my father was responsible for building most of it. No others in the neighborhood had a pond like ours. The Comal Street house was on a corner lot and had nice hedges bordering the yard.

At some point during my early childhood years, in the 1950s, the family moved into what became the first home owned by my mother and my father -- yes -- located at 1908 Emerson Street, a street adjacent to Comal Street. Literally, the house located on Emerson Street was a few steps away from the house on Comal Street, just past two houses away. Our dad had a vision of what the house could become on Emerson Street and he, initially, purchased the lot on which the house would eventually sit.

The reason we moved from the house on Emerson Street in 1969 was due to a government urban renewal program, where we were required to move in favor of what would later become a local university athletic baseball field, which is the current site of baseball games for The University of Texas (at Austin). We lived in the Emerson Street house for about 16 years before being forced by the government to move. We kept the faith – in things hoped for and the evidence of things not yet seen. We believed throughout the transition in being forced to move from one place to another that things would work out fine—and it turned out that we were correct."

The life experiences of the author provided the foundation for and underpinning of the basis upon which the Winners Always Practice Program was developed. Concepts such as continuous improvement, discipline, follow the law, honor, honesty, love, loyalty, respect, trustworthiness were household words and expected standards throughout the family unit and routinely practiced, among other critical behaviors and understandings. The preferred model of how best to communicate and engage with others was always to get along, do things the right way, weapons free, zero bullying of others, and to look for ways to help others – not harm -- and seek the common good over self-interests.

Part One

Winners Always Practice Program (Wapp)

Twenty-one easy-to-address behaviors, practices, qualities and areas of growth and development to win -- in sports and life. By practicing all day everyday each of these categories and components, the chances to win increases in all phases of life, sports, school and for getting along with others within and across race, class and otherwise. Yes, we can all succeed and get along with others, if we wish, by taking time to practice the following well established and accepted behaviors.

Winners Always Practice Program (WAPP) summaries follow, in common terms and examples of biblical passages for alignment and representation of biblical perspective per component, with all passages from The King James Version Study Bible (KJV). Copyright 1988, 2013, 2017 by Liberty University. Publisher: Thomas Nelson, a registered trademark of HarperCollins Christian Publishing, Inc. General Editor: Edward E. Hindson. Some Bible verses were deliberately applied to more than one WAPP concept for reference and alignment.

1. Common sense - Common sense relates to natural tendencies and knowledge based upon routine growth experiences. The

information "bank" to "pull from" or benefit from is common to all, and special training and experiences are not required for reference in determining how best to behave. Or, stated in more common terms, act as if you are smart or well trained and dignified, especially, if others are around or may be affected by your behavior. Always avoid behaving "stupidly" when it is just as easy to behave "smartly." Practice!

➢ *Alignment with Bible Passages:*

"Be not deceived: evil communications corrupt good manners." (1 Corinthians 15: 33)

"But be ye doers of the word, and not hearers only, deceiving your own selves. For if any be a hearer of the word, and not a doer, he is like unto a man beholding his natural face in a glass: For he beholdeth himself, and goeth his way, and straightway forgetteth what manner of man he was. But whoso looketh into the perfect law of liberty, and continueth *therein,* he being not a forgetful hearer, but a doer of the work, this man shall be blessed in his deed." (James 1: 22-25)

"For wisdom *is* better than rubies; and all the things that may be desired are not to be compared to it" (Proverbs 8: 11)

"If thou be wise, thou shalt be wise for thyself: but *if* thou scornest, thou alone shalt bear it." (Proverbs 9: 12)

"Wise *men* lay up knowledge: but the mouth of the foolish *is* near destruction." (Proverbs 10: 14)

"It *is* as sport to a fool to do mischief: but a man of understanding hath wisdom." (Proverbs 10: 23)

"The tongue of the wise useth knowledge aright: but the mouth of fools poureth out foolishness." (Proverbs 15: 2)

"The lips of the wise disperse knowledge: but the heart of the foolish *doeth* not so." (Proverbs 15: 7)

"Folly *is* joy to *him* that *is* destitute of wisdom: but a man of understanding walketh uprightly." (Proverbs 15: 21)

"The heart of the righteous studieth to answer: but the mouth of the wicked poureth out evil things." (Proverbs 15: 28)

Reflection(s): "Let it go!" Let nothing and no one get in the way of your march toward greater success, and always remain goal directed and focused on "winning the game". Make sure all the "dots connect" in a rational manner and avoid blockages of progress by others or yourself. In stressful, tense, and emotional situations, time to practice What to Say, When to Say it, and When to stop talking (WWWST) concepts by using your head, not your mouth until you calm down. Practice: "Let it go!" *These thoughts are used as a foundational statement that appears in each of the principles presented.*

It takes only common sense to understand that the best way to enjoy a high-quality life is to focus on what matters most for good health and well-being for self and family. Therefore, the only time left for interacting with other people is for reaching out to help them, not to distract or bother them in an unwelcomed manner. Whether the setting is in a personal circumstance or in public, it is important to learn to walk away when things appear to get heated, conflictual, or uncomfortable. It is so very disappointing to hear of situations connected to behaviors where someone complains of their "space" being violated, or they complain of someone bothering them in some unwelcomed way. Much of the time it pertains to reports of males being accused of some unacceptable behavior at the high school or college/university level. Sometimes groups are involved in or witness the behavior being reported. Of course, these cases involve women aggressors as well. Stop it before it starts! Stop it! Stop it! Use common sense. Enjoy life in a lane of peace and joy for self, family and help others do the same -- mind your own business. Think, plan, act on what is right, comfortable, and joyful every second of each day.

The author suggests setting up straight talk sessions which include group vignettes, action plays or theatrical activities to illustrate or mimic to our youth various challenges and how best to handle situations which they may encounter. Dramas and other types of simulations can be used to address sensitive issues, such as the following: illicit drugs or alcohol possession or use; weapons showing up on the scene unexpectantly; private matters that may involve intimacy; fighting or other impending altercations and conflicts; lack of school success; depression; problems with peers; and other social-emotional issues of today's youth.

It is common sense to understand that what we think and believe and the actions we take will lead toward or away from the results we expect. For example, if we want to become a high school or college/university graduate, we must enroll in and attend school and complete coursework successfully. If one wants to avoid jail time, follow the law, and do the right things. If a person wishes to become an electrician, complete the requisite training, and so on. It is all about common sense and focusing on doing things at the right time and in the right way. Always remember to compare the risks with the anticipated rewards and minimize, or better to avoid, any risks that may result in problems.

Those who are most successful plan and work hard for the desired outcomes. If you wish to be promoted in your organization, it is commonly understood that the way to best position yourself is to:

- Work hard.
- Demonstrate leadership by example.
- Exhibit good work habits.
- Get along with other employees, show up on time, show willingness to go beyond what is required.
- Show you are dependable.
- Show that the company management can consistently count on you.
- Always have an "own the store" mentality.
- Apply your common sense to every action you take at home or work.

Everybody wants to win, period! The concept of winning applies in multiple angles: sports, work, contracts and more. In life it is more likely than not that one cannot and will not win first place every time desired, no matter how much preparation or degree of intensity in the efforts. There is, however, a difference in not winning first place and defeat. The positive way to look at not winning first place is to analyze what went correctly and what could have gone better and to learn and grow from it and go out and try again. Another way to view not winning is to complain, pout, whine, blame everyone and everything other than those things over which you had control and then quit trying. In that case you are showing signs of being defeated. I enjoyed the days of my competing as an athlete, including my participation in football, basketball and track in junior high school and track and football in high school for only one year and basketball for four years. I served as the high school captain of the basketball team as a senior and played basketball in college. I remain clear that the right attitude to display when you win first place is to show appreciation and that you are humble and grateful for such an honor. I am also clear that there is a right and wrong way to respond to winning and not winning in sports and life, in general.

Winning requires understanding what it is you are competing for as well as degrees of the win. Winning goes beyond winning first place. For example, a track runner in the 100-meter dash who runs a race and comes in last out of eight runners in one race and follows in the next race against the same group and comes in fifth place can rightfully declare himself or herself as winning through making excellent progress. I recall meeting three high school track runners -- and their parents -- at a local university on the running track who were training for the state high school track meet in Texas which was two weeks away. I met one athlete Friday evening and the other two Saturday morning. Each had won first place or second place in the local district and regional track meets in Southeast Texas. They were working hard to be prepared for the state meet and being mentored primarily by their fathers -- thank God for fathers and mothers who will spend their time in this manner. I asked each athlete whether other runners on their school teams had qualified for the state track meet, and the athletes and fathers answered, "Yes". One indicated that she had practiced earlier at the high school the same day. However, after she completed the regularly scheduled practice at the high school, she thought it important to dedicate additional time to practice on her own She was, therefore, going beyond the regular practice session, taking extraordinary measures to prepare for the upcoming state track meet. The other two student athletes also spent time working hard to prepare, beyond the regular high school required practice schedule. In my view, these athletes were already winners, several days prior to the actual state track meet for the state of Texas, sponsored by the Texas University Interscholastic League Organization.

Interestingly, but not surprisingly, the star athletes competing at the high school, college, and professional levels are well acquainted and know the accomplishments of their competitors within the state and on a national basis, ladies, and men. In the eyes of the high school athletes and of their fathers and mothers referenced above, they were not satisfied with just being invited to participate. They were winners who reflected the importance of "always practicing"—fine models of the Winners Always Practice Program. They were also demonstrating common sense; that is, if you want to win, you must practice and not just show up and expect success.

The concept works in adulthood as well. If you want the job or the contract, you must prepare and often outperform others. Therefore, common sense tells you that you may have to devote more time and attention than others or go to school longer in preparation to gain the victory.

There is an additional point to convey regarding the sport of track, and I believe it takes only common sense to address the concern. That is, competitors who compete in running events are not allowed, even, one false start in avoiding disqualification. This rule is preposterous and unreasonable, and it is the only team sport where individuals and entire relay teams are disqualified for such a mistake -- of starting the race too fast. Yet, if you fail to start fast you have much less chance to win the race. In basketball, for example, you can overcome a mistake from start until the final seconds of the contest. It is the same in football, soccer, baseball, softball, and all other team sports. In the past the rule allowed up to two false starts, resulting in some races taking much longer in time to finish. Obviously, the faster you get started affects your ability to finish the race faster than the other runners, especially in the speed races. It is most perplexing that this "no false start" rule is applied even at the level of championship track meets; that is, district, regional, state, and national track meets. The rule is more of a convenience for adults who attend and work at the track meets. It is not enforced in consideration of the student athletes and should be modified to at least allow one false start per racing event prior to disqualification. It is an example of common sense!

The student athlete practices for the entire season and longer for those who practice in advance of the season. The persons charged with management of the start of the races are different in each track meet; thereby, different mannerisms, speed, and cadence in giving the start of the race commands, making it difficult to anticipate how swiftly to get started in the race. If you wait too long to start, you have little to no chance to win, and if you start too fast in anticipating when the race will start -- even one time -- you are disqualified. I can recall in the case of the Texas regional track meets I attended for several years in the Metro-Houston area, the person managing the start of the races was a person who had apparently earned what appeared to be the right for a lifetime commitment to serve as the starter. He was especially slow in his commands and in using the starter pistol for the start of races. Unfortunately, it was routine for individual runners and relay teams to be disqualified for starting their races too fast or making any movements prior to the starting "pistol" being heard. Many, many complained to no avail, and year after year the same shameful and regrettable impact on the youth was experienced. So, who are the advocates for track competitors for changes in this rule? Hopefully, the parents and those track coaches who are serious about coaching in the sport are prime to show such advocacy.

Many high school track coaches consider the coaching assignment to be a secondary assignment, with the primary assignment being that of coaching football or possibly basketball. But even those who may look upon track as a secondary sport, it becomes a priority when faced with the reality of losing the chance to compete in a race due to the runner or relay team facing disqualification because of one false start where the starter is not effective.

I am also concerned about and interested in the rules for disqualification of athletes in the sport of competitive football, due to the act of what is commonly referred to "targeting" -- direct hit by the helmet of a player against an opponent when the player lowers the head to initiate and contact his helmet against the opposing player. The implementation of the penalty for such an action results in a penalty of 15 yards and disqualification of the offending player. The rule puts the defensive players at a disadvantage because of the difficulty of being able to make the tackle against the opponent while moving full speed as that player on offense is also moving full speed. Of course, it makes sense to implement policies for ensuring safety of the players. Imposing the penalty of 15 yards against the offending player's team is enough to make the point of the need to avoid direct helmet hits. It does not make sense that for the full course of the remainder of a football game (which by nature of the way the game is played involves hitting each other), that a rule would be in place not only to punish the player for hitting a certain way, but to "kick the player out of the rest of the game", regardless of the point in the game the infraction occurs. There are many ways to emphasize the intended points, such as to increase the penalty for the infraction to 20 yards instead of 15 and leave the offending player in the game or increase the penalty to more than 15 yards and remove the player for the remainder of that quarter in which the infraction occurs -- which means the player would be ejected only if the infraction occurs during the fourth quarter of the game.

Getting back to common sense, in general. It is common sense to know that everyone deserves and expects to be treated with dignity and respect. Yet, it is far too routine to find conflict around issues of one's race, level of income or class in human interactions. It is common sense and fact that when a child is born, intellect is not determined based upon race or environment. Things happen from the first day of birth through an accumulation of events, level of care and attention and environment which contribute to molding intellectual growth and development. Therefore, the so-called gaps in achievement, as manifested in test scores among races and other child groupings occur following birth, based upon several factors, such as:

- A child's circumstances -- environmental conditions and access to proper health care.

- Whether plentiful reading materials are available with consistent opportunities to read and having someone read to them.
- Exposure to the arts.
- Sophistication and routine use of appropriate grammar and high-level verbal and visual cues and language in communication among adults and older children.
- Local and not so local travel experiences.
- Proper nutrition.
- Models on the importance of academic and social advancement, and more.

In growing up while living on Emerson Street in Austin, the other neighborhood children and I walked to visit nearby neighborhoods and children of our same age group. The differences were stark in comparisons of wealth and access to opportunities between our immediate neighborhood group and the children from the more affluent areas of the community. We got along well, and communication was friendly. The visits, however, stopped at the doorsteps of our homes, seldom including an invitation or interest in going inside. Yet, we all sought the same things in terms of joy and quality of life. There were more similarities than differences in our character and interests in happiness and being successful in school and other areas of life. We did well to navigate our paths to enjoy the similarities and did not allow differences in race and class or income levels dictate our ability to get along.

How many times during a given day do you see a situation where someone fails to use common sense? Think about it. Pay attention and you can recognize multiple examples all around, where a person would have only needed to stop and think before acting to avoid problems. For example:

- Automobile accidents.
- A person falls off a ladder or house roof.
- Engaging in non-marital and/or unprotected sex, resulting in pregnancy or disease.
- Assaulting or taking advantage of others, especially children in any manner or form.

- Cooking and going to sleep or another room while the burner is still on and not monitored.
- Stuffing yourself with food multiple times a day and not exercising.
- Going to work or participating in a sports contest tired and not resting the evening before.
- Participating in a big meeting at work or sports contest without studying the requisite materials.
- Showing up for a big meeting at work or sports contest without taking time to practice beforehand.
- Using credit cards beyond the ability to pay.
- Gun accidents.
- Resisting science-based health notifications such as wearing a mask during a virus pandemic.
- Driving or riding in an automobile with illegal weapons or drugs.
- Posting pictures and negative comments on social media and not expecting repercussions.
- Being lazy on the job or team and later expecting a promotion or more playing time.
- Negative attitude and unfriendly with co-workers or teammates and wonder why unliked and not respected.
- You share a "juicy" private or personal story or picture with a friend or colleague directly or during a remote/virtual conference experience and wonder if the information will be shared widely with others.
- You break the law and get angry when caught.
- Showing up to take a test without first studying the material.
- You show crude and unprofessional conduct in front of children and expect them not to copy.

Practice!

Reader - Think; Share; Reflect: _____

_____

_____

2. Continuous improvement - No one is perfect, and everyone can and should strive to improve. Part of the human growth and development experience is that natural changes occur over which we have no control. Regarding those things over which we do have control, it is imperative to plan for and take advantage of opportunities to improve, within and across all forms of knowledge and conduct. It is safe to say that a person is on the incline in growth and development or in decline, as nothing in the human existence remains the same, over time. Never, ever give up or quit. Practice!

➢ *Alignment with Bible Passages*:

"But let every man prove his own work, and then shall he have rejoicing in himself alone, and not in another. For every man shall bear his own burden." (Galatians 6: 4-5)

"Give *instruction* to a wise *man*, and he will be yet wiser: teach a just *man*, and he will increase in learning." (Proverbs: 9: 9)

"Whoso loveth instruction loveth knowledge: but he that hateth reproof *is* brutish." (Proverbs 12: 1)

"Train up a child in the way he should go: and when he is old, he will not depart from it." Proverbs 22: 6)

"I can do all things through Christ which strengtheneth me." (Phillipians 4: 13)

"But they that wait upon the LORD shall renew *their* strength; they shall mount up with wings as eagles; they shall run, and not be weary; *and* they shall walk, and not faint." (Isaiah 40: 31)

"For that which I do I allow not: for what I would, that do I not; but what I hate, that do I. If then I do that which I would not, I consent unto the law that *it is* good. Now then it is no more I that do it, but sin that dwelleth in me." (Romans 7:15-17)

"I will instruct thee and teach thee in the way which thou shalt go: I will guide thee with mine eye." (Psalm 32: 8)

"When I was a child, I spake as a child, I understood as a child, I thought as a child: but when I became a man, I put away childish things." (1 Corinthians 13: 11)

"But let patience have *her* perfect work, that ye may be perfect and entire, wanting nothing. If any of you lack wisdom, let him ask of God, that giveth to all *men* literally, and upbraideth not; and it shall be given him." (James 1: 4-5)

Reflection(s): "Let it go!" Let nothing and no one get in the way of your march toward greater success, and always remain goal directed and focused on "winning the game". Make sure all the "dots connect" in a rational manner and avoid blockages of progress by others or yourself. In stressful, tense, and emotional situations, time to practice WWWST concepts by using your head, not your mouth until you calm down. Practice: "Let it go!"

There is no easy ride toward victory; you must work for it. Whether the activity is reading, delivering speeches or presentations, working on the job, riding a bicycle or other physical activities, the more you practice, the opportunity for improvement increases. Stop practicing and you decline in skills and reduce, if not eliminate, the potential for improvement. "Use it or lose it."

I can recall numerous stories of the "march toward excellence", going back to childhood, on how individuals, in general, and athletic teams moved from the performance level of mediocre or average to the "top of the class" in their sport. Examples follow:

- High school and college classmates who devoted time after school, weekends and summers practicing their sport, reading, and studying, moving on to win scholarships for college and contracts in professional sports and toward successful careers, spanning all forms of disciplines.

- Perennial athletics and professional championship teams who win and compete successfully year in and out at the high school, college, and professional levels in all sports. How does this happen? They work hard at continuous improvement, and they focus on teamwork and achieving their mission -- not some of the time, but all the time.

- Artists such as Itzhak Perlman, a famous and phenomenally successful violinist and conductor. I had the pleasure to meet him and enjoy one of his performances at Lamar University in Beaumont, Texas. He was most humble throughout the performance and in conversation about his remarkable success and how practicing made the greatest difference in his rise to the "top" as a violinist. Perlman, who was born in Tel Aviv, contracted polio at a young age but did not let that stop him in his march toward success. When I met him, he used a scooter and crutches to aide in his mobility but made no excuses and did not complain about the relevant challenges in movement. When asked about what had made the greatest difference in his success, beyond the encouragement from his parents, he pointed to how much he practiced, practiced, practiced to continuously improve in his skills.

- I recall playing racquetball games at The University of Texas at Austin against a lady who was much younger than I and shorter in height. She won each game by large margins, and it was an embarrassing experience. In leaving the gym she reminded me to think of the "glass as half full" and not "half empty" and that practicing will make the difference in improving my skills in the sport. She was right, and in time upon a lot more practice, I improved my skills in every aspect of the game, including thinking strategically about where to hit the ball and how to keep the ball low in hitting it off the wall, making it harder for the opponent to respond.

- I was honored and pleased to attend a ballet performance of "super" ballerina, Misty Copeland, in Costa Mesa, California in 2015: <u>The Nutcracker</u>. Ms. Copeland was the first African American dancer named as a principal dancer with the American Ballet Theatre. My wife, Carolyn, and I enjoyed the pleasure of meeting and speaking briefly with her backstage following the program. All performers did an excellent job, and Ms. Copeland was outstanding in performing her role in the production. Coincidentally, we had enjoyed lunch at a restaurant near the theatre -- Segerstrom Center for The Arts--and met some of the youth who also were part of the program. They explained that they were members of the team traveling and performing as part of the American Ballet Theatre program and were excited to perform with Misty. The youth and Misty Copeland spoke of and demonstrated in their performance the importance of practicing to perfect the skills required to perform successfully.

Think of the best performers for any activity or job and ask the question of how they attained the skills for achieving at that level. No doubt, they practiced, practiced, practiced, and exhibited extraordinary passion for achievement. This point holds true in sports and every other activity. The lazy and those who refuse to put in the time and demonstrate the commitment and passion for continuous improvement cannot achieve at the best of anything. This point is transferable regardless of the activity. In one real-life, important example that affects the growth and development of children and quality of life: reading, reading, reading consistently several hours per day results in improved reading skills, including comprehension, recognizing, and understanding words and increasing knowledge.

Never give up. So often the victory is just beyond the temptation to quit. In fact, one of the enemies of victory is not to try at all. It has been said that you cannot get to second base in baseball if you keep your foot on first base. Likewise, if you want to know what is in the book, you must first open it, and so on. This logic works in all fields or endeavors. For example, as education leader and human and civil rights advocate, I have worked hard to ensure that children enjoy learning in facilities which are appropriate and comparable to those considered to be among the finest. All our children deserve the nicest environments to learn in regardless of which neighborhood they live in and their zip code. I have made deliberate attempts as an educator to go beyond the words in my commitment on making sure students have access to appropriate school facilities.

The challenges may be great for achieving something extraordinary, but that is no excuse not to try to succeed. Examples follow:

- Austin, Texas - The University of Texas at Austin -- The completion of the doctorate was an amazing opportunity, including the networking among the school cohort group of students who had come from varied, diverse backgrounds and experiences. It took several tries before I was accepted into the program. But I did not allow the challenges for getting into the school affect the outcome of my getting out and earning the Doctor of Philosophy degree. I was proud to graduate with straight "A" s in my coursework, including a perfect score in the two-day writing examination finals before graduation. Such success was only possible because I had worked hard and practiced each day on continuous improvement. Practice!

- Birmingham, Alabama -- The school district had not built a new high school in more than 30 years upon my selection as superintendent. Working with the City of Birmingham and State of Alabama officials, the school board and I set about replacing the original Carver High School with the George Washington Carver High School for Health Professions, Engineering and Technology. We started with the vision for building this new school and several others, while renovating campuses where renovation was sufficient. Upgrading technology in all schools was also a major part of the plan. We were successful in getting it all done! We kept the faith and did not give up.

- Port Arthur, Texas – The community passed a bond issue which included providing funds for building a new high school prior to my tenure as superintendent. Several years later, no movement was made for achieving the vision because of confusion and disagreements about the intended site of the new building. After years of delay, the impact of inflation blocked the opportunity to proceed, as the architectural drawings were already completed, but the funds available were insufficient for completing the project. I was fortunate upon my selection as superintendent to provide administrative leadership in coordination with the school board to determine the appropriate school site and for raising the additional bond funds through approval of the community to get the job done. We were successful in building the beautiful Memorial High School. We did not give up and, by working together, we were able to improve the educational environment for the children for this school and all others in the school district.

In what areas of your life are you working on improving? Remember, if not working to improve, you are operating in an attitude of decline. Think about it; does any of the items listed below align with those areas which you believe you could or should work on to improve? It is never too late to start; now is as good a time as any.

- Reading and writing -- At least 20 minutes per day and targeting 60 or more.
- Exercising, including walking, or running a minimum of 10,000 steps per day.
- Living a healthy lifestyle, including eating, and drinking routines and securing sufficient daily rest.
- Listening carefully to others in conversation and not interrupting.
- Practicing knowing what to say, when to say it and when to stop talking.
- Thinking about and acting on helping others and serving the "common good" or team over self.
- Looking for ways to be nice to other people, cheering them up over pushing to get your way.
- Taking time beyond being told to prepare and practice before a meeting or team sports contest.
- Dedicating sufficient time for meditation, rest, and relaxation.

- Taking time to demonstrate appreciation, concern, love, and support for family and teammates or work associates.
- Focusing while driving and not texting or allowing distractions.
- In stressful times demonstrating self-discipline and self-respect and not "going along to get along".
- Working at improving skills at the job and sports activities.
- "Standing up" for right over wrong, even when the faced with possible revenge or retaliation.

Practice!
Reader - Think; Share; Reflect: _____

_____

_____

3. Discipline - Self-discipline is about making choices that are controlled by only one person, that is you! It is one of the most important decisions and, yet, too often one of the most challenging to manage. When managed effectively you stay out of trouble and avoid being confronted with problems and circumstances which can easily become a distraction and block progress toward happiness and well-being. Practice!

➤ *Alignment with Bible Passages:*

"Now no chastening for the present seemeth to be joyous, but grievous: nevertheless afterward it yieldeth the peaceable fruit of righteousness unto them which are exercised thereby." (Hebrews 12: 11)

"Obey them that have the rule over you, and submit yourselves: for they watch for your souls, as they that must give account, that they may do it with joy, and not with grief: for that *is* unprofitable for you." (Hebrews 13: 17)

"He shall die without instruction; and in the greatness of his folly he shall go astray." (Proverbs 5: 23)

"WHOSO loveth instruction loveth knowledge: but he that hateth reproof *is* brutish. A good *man* obtaineth favour of the LORD: but a man of wicked devices will he condemn. A man shall not be established by wickedness: but the root of the righteous shall not be moved. A virtuous woman *is* a crown to her husband: but she that maketh ashamed *is* as rottenness in his bones. The thoughts of the righteous *are* right: *but* the counsels of the wicked *are* deceit." (Proverbs 12: 1-5)

"He that refuseth instruction despiseth his own soul: but he that heareth reproof getteth understanding." (Proverbs 15: 32)

"Love not sleep, lest thou come to poverty; open thine eyes, *and* thou shalt be satisfied with bread." (Proverbs 20: 13)

"Correct thy son, and he shall give thee rest; yea, he shall give delight unto thy soul. Where *there is* no vision, the people perish: but he that keepeth the law, happy *is* he." (Proverbs 29: 17-18)

"Children, obey your parents in the LORD: for this is right. Honour Thy Father And Mother; which is the first commandment with promise. That it may be well with thee, and thou mayest live long on the earth. And, ye fathers, provoke not your children to wrath: but bring them up in the nurture and admonition of the LORD." (Ephesians 6: 1-4)

"But they that wait upon the LORD shall renew *their* strength; they shall mount up with wings as eagles; they shall run, and not be weary; *and* they shall walk and not faint." (Isaiah 40: 31)

"Know ye not that they which run in a race run all, but one receiveth the prize? So run, that ye may obtain. And every man that striveth for the mastery is temperate in all things. Now they *do it* to obtain a corruptible crown; but we an

18

incorruptible. I therefore so run, not as uncertainly; so fight I, not as one that beateth the air; But I keep under my body, and bring *it* into subjection: lest that by any means, when I have preached to others, I myself should be a castaway." (1 Corinthians 9: 24-27)

Reflection(s): "Let it go!" Let nothing and no one get in the way of your march toward greater success, and always remain goal directed and focused on "winning the game". Make sure all the "dots connect" in a rational manner and avoid blockages of progress by others or yourself. In stressful, tense, and emotional situations, time to practice WWWST concepts by using your head, not your mouth until you calm down. Practice: "Let it go!"

Self-discipline is much easier to think and talk about than to demonstrate. It is so much easier because making the right choice may mean balancing or rejecting the decision on what we may want with the decision on what may be better for us or what we may need. It is always about making choices -- good ones or poor ones that propel our paths toward victory, winning or losing. Discipline spans across and within the other components of the WAPP and can make all the difference in the world in a positive way when the right decision is made. When the wrong or questionable decision is made, it can result in something negative. Making a choice can be so much easier than we sometimes make it. Think about it. For example, in deciding on healthy food choices, you can eat a carrot rather than a potato chip if you feel the urge to eat something with a crunchy sound. On another healthy lifestyle choice, most of us can walk a mile for a portion of the day just as easily as deciding to sit on the couch all day and getting little to no exercise that day. You can choose to drink a bottle of water just as easily as deciding to drink a can or bottle of soda or alcohol. And it is reasonable to believe that many of those things that otherwise may be important to avoid in large amounts may be useful in moderation.

Is it not just as easy to smile as it is to frown during a conversation? What about displaying an advent attitude for giving over pushing to take for oneself or to selfishly focus on self over giving or helping others? Is it not just as easy to be nice as it is to be not so nice or to be mean? If the idea is to win the game or win the contract, it makes more sense to practice with the team and to develop and follow the game plan than to miss practice or not to plan or practice at all. Think of the responsibility to go to a meeting on a workday or go to school during a school day. It makes more sense to go than to look for excuses not to go. Winners not only go where they are expected and required or when the team is counting on them, they act beyond ordinary and excel to achieve at the highest levels. Winners think and act like champions, all the time, which means they also demonstrate a sense of pride and dignity and self-discipline.

During any day, a person routinely is faced with making numerous decisions about what to do. Some choices are easier to deal with than others. In some situations, the decisions hold life or death consequences in the balance. One easy decision for all is never to drink and drive, and never to allow a friend to drink and drive while under the influence of alcohol. Of course, as importantly never use illegal drugs or allow a friend to use illegal drugs and drive an automobile. In self-discipline it is not only an acceptable practice, but also highly appropriate to think about each decision, whether the decision comports with your intended, well thought out strategy or plan for self-discipline. If you have no plan or strategy in place, today is a good day to start in designing one.

Self-discipline is at play when a person decides whether to report on time or late to work or a team practice session. Here is a place where commitment may be applied, that is, commitment to self and others that you will uphold your promise to help achieve the victory for the place of work or sports or another team. Self-discipline is also at play when a person makes the decision to prepare to succeed for self and team -- taking time to rest and eating in appropriate measures, preparing for, and completing all assignments fully and on time and communicating while using active listening skills over pushing just to get your way. It is always about the common good or what is best for the team; no letter "I" in the word or meaning of the term "team". Practice!

Reader - Think; Share; Reflect: _____

_____

_____

4. Focus - It is so easy to set goals and, yet, much more difficult to focus and set plans for and take the actions that are necessary to achieve them. Focusing entails controlling thoughts and actions to address with laser like attention on what matters the most. To focus is also not allowing distractions that may delay or prevent the outcomes desired. You can always find some reason not to focus and many better reasons to focus and maintain it, regardless of the temptations to do otherwise. Practice!

   ➤ *Alignment with Bible Passages:*

   "Let thine eyes look right on, and let thine eyelids look straight before thee." (Proverbs 4: 25)

   "Finally, brethren, whatsoever things are true, whatsoever things *are* honest, whatsoever things *are* just, whatsoever things *are* pure, whatsoever things *are* lovely, whatsoever things *are* of good report; if *there* be any virtue, and if *there be* any praise, think on these things." (Philippians 4: 8)

   "When I was a child, I spake like a child, I understood as a child, I thought as a child: but when I became a man, I put away childish things." (1 Corinthians 13: 11)

   "For the *kingdom of heaven is* as a man traveling into a far country, *who* called his own servants, and delivered unto them his goods. And unto one he gave five talents, to another two, and to another one, to every man according to his several ability; and straightway took his journey. Then he that had received the five talents went and traded with the same, and made *them* other five talents. And likewise he that *had received* two, he also gained other two. But he that had received one went and digged in the earth, and hid his lord's money." (Matthew 25: 14-18)

   "And the LORD answered me, and said, Write the vision, and make *it* plain upon tables, that he may run that readeth

Dr. Johnny E. Brown

it. For the vision *is* yet for an appointed time, but at the end it shall speak, and not lie: though it tarry, wait for it; because it will surely come, it will not tarry." (Habakkuk 2: 2-3)

"Brethen, I count not myself to have apprehended: but *this* one thing I *do*, forgetting those things which are behind, and reaching forth unto those things which are before." (Philippians 3: 13)

"Now faith is the substance of things hoped for, the evidence of things not seen." (Hebrews 11: 1)

"And I sent messengers unto them, saying, I *am* doing great work, so that I cannot come down: why should the work cease, whilst I leave it, and come down to you?" (Nehemiah 6: 3)

"Set your affection on things above, not on things on the earth." (Colossians 3: 2)

"Whatsoever thy hand findeth to do, do *it* with thy might; for *there is* no work, nor device, nor knowledge, nor wisdom, in the grave, whither thou goest." (Ecclesiastes 9: 10)

Reflection(s): "Let it go!" Let nothing and no one get in the way of your march toward greater success, and always remain goal directed and focused on "winning the game". Make sure all the "dots connect" in a rational manner and avoid blockages of progress by others or yourself. In stressful, tense, and emotional situations, time to practice WWWST concepts by using your head, not your mouth until you calm down. Practice: "Let it go!"

It is especially important to focus, and it is your decision whether to maintain a positive attitude, especially in stressful situations. The only difference is your attitude which you alone can manage and control. In fact, it is a waste of time focusing on those things over which you have little to no control, and it is essential to recognize that your attitude is one of those things you do control, 100% of the time. It is far better to maintain a positive attitude and treat others with a sense of hospitality and not ever allow yourself to drift into a lane of any appearance of being mean or "messing with people". Always remain focused on achieving the victory you set out to achieve and avoid distractions which may impede your progress. Look at champions of any sport or any avenue of life and what you will find are those individuals who have set goals and objectives and work hard to achieve them. They also demonstrate the ability to avoid those things that are not important. They set their minds on what matters and zoom in with laser like focus. Winners know that the path to victory is often not an easy one. Note, it is not coincidental that those who win consistently are repeaters in winning, such as the Kansas City Chiefs in professional football or Alabama and Clemson Universities in college football. Other notable examples include Simone Biles in gymnastics, Michael Jordan, Kareem Abdul Jabbar and Kobe Bryant in professional basketball. Whether the game or sport or avenue of life is about victory by an individual or team or company, the same people often repeat as winners. They believe in themselves and their plan of operations. The indicators of success and winning strategies are posted and adhered to. They work hard for the victory, and they focus on doing the little things and big things to "play to win". You cannot be almost focused and win. Close is just not good enough.

Think of the many scenarios where focusing matters, whether in sports or work or day-to-day activities. It is extremely easy to become distracted or lazy and mindless for the moment. Yet, think about it; it may take only a moment of losing focus that can result in a life-threatening circumstance:

- While driving.
- Cooking.
- Delivering an important speech.
- Taking a paper-pencil test.
- Completing a work assignment.
- Playing in a game, such as basketball, football or soccer, and the ball is tossed or kicked in your direction -- lose focus and you, literally, can lose the game or, even, a life.

True, it does take effort to focus, but it is necessary for success. I can recall, for example, in numerous television and radio shows where I participated in conversations with the hosts and others, in some cases where there were thousands in the listening and viewing audience. I took extraordinary care to listen and make comments that were appropriate to the situation -- excuses and mistakes not acceptable. A few memorable instances follow that required strict focus on my part: a nationally televised program on the Cable News Network (CNN) regarding the Dekalb County Schools' student dress code; and another livestream program on the importance of reading, along with the United States Department of Education Secretary of Education, Richard Riley. The program was a nationally televised discussion on the importance of emphasizing literacy in educating our children. I also participated in numerous locally televised programs and radio and print media interviews during my career. I always tried to focus intently each moment of the interview. In another example, I was invited to meet with the President of the United States, George W. Bush in the White House regarding the pending legislation for the "No Child Left Behind" national schools accountability program. There were only 20 or so participants invited to participate, including State Department of Education Commissioners and Secretaries of Education for various states and a couple of local school superintendents, including myself. Also included were a few governors, the United States Secretary of Homeland Security, and many media representatives at the post-meeting news conference. This was no time to be distracted or having a wandering mindset. I had to maintain focus to be relevant in the conversation and to best serve the children I was there to represent. I also recall the many presentations I delivered for hundreds of people and even when the audience was small, I was clear on the importance of focusing, listening, and responding with purpose.

When a person is playing in a game like football or basketball, track, tennis, golf, swimming, hockey, soccer, and other sports, it is important to think "team" over "self" and to focus during every play: shooting a free throw, or catching a forward pass, or hitting the golf ball, or accepting a pass in soccer, and more. For example, consider what happened at the end of a national football league football game,

December 26, 2020 where a team scored a field goal, putting the team ahead by two points with only 19 seconds left in the game, and almost miraculously the team ended up losing by one point. Once the team scored the field goal putting their team ahead, they kicked the ball to the opposing team – again, with only 19 seconds left. A player on defense made the huge mistake of grabbing the opposing quarterback's facemask, spinning him around, resulting in a 15 penalty, which was marked off at the end of the play -- which included completion of a long forward pass, putting the opposing team in place for a forty-four-yard field goal. That play put the opposing team ahead by one point. Lack of focus; lack of proper technique; avoidable mistake, and the team which had just gone ahead in the game with a field goal with only 19 seconds left in the game lost the game. Of course, one play or one mistake does not mean the rest of the plays during the game were not important but, in this case, the mistake was a critical miscue that could have been avoided if only the player had focused better on the situation at hand. The importance of focusing holds true for settings such as business and church meetings. Focus! Play to win the game and to succeed. Practice!

Reader - Think; Share; Reflect: _____

_____

_____

5. Follow Law - Laws exist for a reason: to protect all from harm, promote democracy and support us all as we seek to enjoy the "common good" and better quality of life. Do what you are supposed to do and not what you are not to do. Always keep the brain "open", and keep the thoughts and actions directed toward advantages for and reasons to follow all laws whether local, state or nationally generated. There is always a possibility of being caught, thereby, bringing negative attention toward you along with penalties which can derail or ruin the "road" to winning on and off the playing field or court. Remember, in the "world" of current technology, officials can find out all kinds of information through review of records from cameras, cell phones, credit cards and banking records. Sooner or later when

you fail to follow the law, you will be caught and will face the consequences of your actions. Practice!

➢ *Alignment with Bible Passages:*

"For not the hearers of the law *are* just before God, but the doers of the law shall be justified." (Romans 2: 13)

"Let every soul be subject unto the higher powers. For there is no power but of God: the powers that be are ordained of God . . . Render therefore to all their dues: tribute to whom tribute *is due*; custom to whom custom; fear to whom fear; honour to whom honour." (Romans 13: 1; 7)

"Put them in mind to be subject to principalities and powers, to obey magistrates, to be ready to every good work." (Titus 3: 1)

"*Is* the law then against the promises of God? God forbid: for if there had been a law given which could have given life, verily righteousness should have been by the law. But the scripture hath concluded all under sin, that the promise by faith of Jesus Christ might be given to them that believe. But before faith came, we were kept under the law, shut up unto the faith which should afterwards be revealed. Wherefore the law was our schoolmaster to *bring us* unto Christ, that we might be justified by faith" (Galatians 3: 21-24)

"But the fruit of the Spirit is love, joy, peace, long-suffering, gentleness, goodness, faith, Meekness, temperance: against such there is no law." (Galatians 5: 22-23)

"They that forsake the law praise the wicked: but such as keep the law contend with them. Evil men understand not judgment: but they that seek the LORD understand all *things*. Better *is* the poor that walketh in his uprightness, than *he that is* perverse *in his* ways, though he *be* rich. Whoso keepeth the law *is* a wise son: but he that is a companion of riotous *men* shameth his father." (Proverbs 28: 4 - 7)

"But the fearful, and unbelieving, and the abominable, and murderers, and whoremongers, and sorcerers and idolators, and all liars, shall have their part in the lake which burneth with fire and brimstone: which *is* the second death." (Revelation 21: 8)

"Blessed *is* the man that walketh not in the counsel of the ungodly, nor standeth in the way of sinners, nor sitteth in the seat of the scornful. But his delight *is* in the law of the LORD; and in his law doth he meditate day and night. And he shall be like a tree planted by the rivers of water, that bringeth forth his fruit in his season; his leaf also shall not wither; and whatsoever he doeth shall prosper. The ungodly *are* not so; but *are* like the chaff which the wind driveth away. Therefore, the ungodly shall not stand in the judgment, nor sinners in the congregation of the righteous. For the LORD knoweth the way of the righteous: but the way of the ungodly shall perish." (Psalm 1: 1 – 6)

"Whosoever committeth sin transgresseth also the law: for sin is the transgression of the law." (1 John 3: 4)

"But whoso looketh into the perfect law of liberty, and continueth *therein,* he being not a forgetful hearer, but a doer of the work, this man shall be blessed in his deed." (James 1: 25)

Reflection(s): "Let it go!" Let nothing and no one get in the way of your march toward greater success, and always remain goal directed and focused on "winning the game". Make sure all the "dots connect" in a rational manner and avoid blockages of progress by others or yourself. In stressful, tense, and emotional situations, time to practice WWWST concepts by using your head, not your mouth until you calm down. Practice: "Let it go!"

No excuses acceptable; follow the law, period! Of course, there may be instances which arise where disputes or lack of understandings may lead to legal disputes. And everyone is prone to make mistakes. Yet, where possible, better to keep it simple and do what is easily the right thing to do. When you know the law or question whether something is or is not lawful, err each time on the side of caution and avoidance, so as not to take the chance of your actions being out of line with the law. Do only those things which you know and believe are the right things to do. Look out for your neighbor in helping somebody over doing that which may be harmful to self or others.

Happiness and joy are generally not achievable when contemplating or taking actions which may result in pain and suffering for yourself or others. After all, the primary reason that we have laws in place is to serve justice in favor of the common good -- that includes for you and all others. The consequences for doing the wrong thing in breaking the law are bothersome for the companies or victims affected by the crime and, ultimately, for the perpetrator when apprehended. It is not worth it to even think criminality, let alone commit crimes. It is easy to rationalize in your thinking the possible benefits if not caught with the consequences one faces if apprehended. The chances are greater that you will be caught -- then, again, everyone affected is harmed, including you and your family and the persons targeted by your illegal actions. It is just not worth it. Follow the law every day of life. Also, always remember this simple rule: "Don't mess with other people, their property or their money", and life is, therefore, better for you and all others around you. True winners make wise choices and among the wisest of choices one can make is to follow the law -- do what you are supposed to do and not what you are not.

Think about the calm and pleasant comfort of enjoying the freedom to come and go, stay, or leave, deciding how to spend your free time and with whom. Such calm or serenity in life is earned by doing the right things and controlling one's actions. Break the law and you risk losing those privileges and many more, and it is your choice. Follow the law, period!

And always keep in mind the thought: "<u>Leave other people alone, except to help them</u>!" Practice!

28

Reader - Think; Share; Reflect: _____

_____

_____

6. Healthy lifestyle (no alcohol, drugs, eat right & exercise) - Being healthy is directly affected and driven by lifestyle and choices about eating, drinking, exercising, resting, and intake of substances. Attitude makes a difference realizing, for example, that expending the energy for a smile is far less difficult to develop than to develop a frown, and the impact is more healthful. To smile and seek happiness and acting out such an emotion is a good idea. Remember, how you live your life is your decision and none is more important than to choose to live a healthy lifestyle. Practice!

➤ *Alignment with Bible Passages*:

"Be not wise in thine own eyes: fear the LORD, and depart from evil. It shall be health to thy navel, and marrow to thy bones. Honour the LORD with thy substance, and with the first fruits of all thine increase." *(Proverbs 3: 7-9)*

"A sound heart *is* the life of the flesh: but envy the rottenness of the bones." (Proverbs 14: 30)

"A merry heart doeth good *like* a medicine: but a broken spirit drieth the bones." (Proverbs 17: 22)

"Be not among winebibbers; among riotous eaters of flesh: For the drunkard and the glutton shall come to poverty: and drowsiness shall clothe *a man* with rags." (Proverbs 23: 20-21)

"He giveth power to the faint; and to *them that have* no might he increaseth strength. Even the youths shall faint and be weary, and the young men shall utterly fall: But they that wait upon the LORD shall renew *their* strength; they shall mount up with wings as eagles; they shall run, and not be weary; *and* they shall walk, and not faint." (Isaiah 40: 29-31)

"Beloved, I wish above all things that thou mayest prosper and be in health, even as thy soul prospereth." (3 John 1: 2)

"And God said, Behold, I have given you every herb bearing seed, which *is* upon the face of all the earth, and every tree, in the which *is* the fruit of a tree yielding seed; to you it shall be for meat. And to every beast of the earth, and to every fowl of the air, and to every thing that creepeth upon the earth, wherein *there* is life, I *have given* every green herb for meat: and it was so." (Genesis 1: 29-30)

"Him that *is* weak in the faith receive ye, *but* not to doubtful disputations. For one believeth that he may eat all things: another, who is weak, eateth herbs. Let not him that eateth despise him that eateth not; and let not him which eateth not judge him that eateth: for God hath received him." (Romans 14: 1-3)

"Therefore I say unto you, Take no thought for your life, what ye shall eat, or what ye shall drink; nor yet for your body, what ye shall put on. Is not the life more than meat, and the body than raiment? Behold the fowls of the air: for they sow not, neither do they reap, nor gather into barns; yet your heavenly Father feedeth them. Are ye not much better than they." (Matthew 6: 25-26)

"For bodily exercise profiteth little: but godliness is profitable unto all things, having promise of the life that now is, and of that which is to come." (1 Timothy 4: 8)

Reflection(s): "Let it go!" Let nothing and no one get in the way of your march toward greater success, and always remain goal directed and focused on "winning the game". Make sure all the "dots connect" in a rational manner and avoid blockages of progress by others or yourself.

In stressful, tense, and emotional situations, time to practice WWWST concepts by using your head, not your mouth until you calm down. Practice: "Let it go!"

Start today if you have not already figured this out, eat healthy foods, including fruits and vegetables, and eat other foods in moderation and exercise daily. Complicated concept, no -- not at all. Yet, it is apparent from the data and observations all around us that far too many of us do not follow this simple rule. I recall a conversation with an employee at an airport luggage check-in area where the gentleman said that he had waited until he was 60 years old to decide to start eating fruits and vegetables. Too late? No, not at all; better late than never. But much better had he and all of us been mindful to start at infancy and maintained the standard through childhood and young adulthood and beyond. It can be done and is necessary for the best possible quality of life and well-being. This is an area where making good choices makes a major difference in whether a person wins for high quality of life or positions oneself for a lifestyle that ensures a path toward problems that are avoidable.

Consider the training regimen and eating and exercise routines of the best athletes during the time of their participation in action sports. The most successful of them eat healthy foods with set schedules and routines, and they exercise, often pushing themselves beyond ordinary for the best results. Some even go so far as hiring nutritionists and trainers for organizing menus and practice schedules. The term "discipline" comes to mind here. Why? Because part of any plan for success requires discipline and psychological edge. If it were easy and anyone could do it, there would be more limited separation between those who succeed and those who do not. Yet, it is possible for each person to enjoy victory in lifestyle and better health by simply making the right decisions and maintaining the discipline as needed to eat properly. That means regular helpings of fruits and vegetables and not going heavy on meats and fried foods and by implementing a schedule of vigorous exercise. Of course, all should get an adequate amount of rest each day and avoid the use of smoking and other drugs and alcohol. Among numerous other important factors for winning in life and enjoying a high quality of life, excellent health practices translate strongly as an especially important factor. Choices, choices, choices. In the case of health and well-being, making the right choices may mean the difference of enjoying a happy, high quality lifestyle or the opposite. Practice!

Reader - Think; Share; Reflect: _____

_____

_____

7. Honor (think and act your best with integrity and character) – Everyone has a name. That "good name" represents your family, self, and history -- past and future. The best way to protect that "good name" is to think and act with integrity and strong character. Such behavior is expected and preferred in all circles of life across the world, characterized by carrying oneself and treating others with respect and dignity and in accordance with the law and "high" moral character. Practice!

➢ *Alignment with Bible Passages*:

"He that walketh uprightly walketh surely: but he that perverteth his ways shall be known." (Proverbs 10: 9)

"The integrity of the upright shall guide them: but the perverseness of transgressors shall destroy them." (Proverbs 11: 3)

"The righteousness of the perfect shall direct his way: but the wicked shall fall by his own wickedness. The righteousness of the upright shall deliver them: but transgressors shall be taken in *their own* naughtiness." (Proverbs 11: 5-6)

"Better *is* the poor that walketh in his uprightness, than *he that is* perverse *in his* ways, though he *be* rich." (Proverbs 28: 6)

"He that is faithful in that which is least is faithful also in much: and he that is unjust in the least is unjust also in much." (Luke 16: 10)

"Finally, brethren, whatsoever things *are* true, whatsoever things *are* honest, whatsoever things *are* just, whatsoever things *are* pure, whatsoever things *are* lovely, whatsoever things *are* of good report; if *there be* any virtue, and if *there be* any praise, think on these things." (Philippians 4: 8)

"And as ye would that men should do to you, do ye also to them likewise." (Luke 6:31)

"And hath not oppressed any *but* hath restored to the debtor his pledge, hath spoiled none by violence, hath given his bread to the hungry, and hath covered the naked with a garment . . . Hath walked in my statutes, and hath kept my judgements, to deal truly; he *is* just, he shall surely live, saith the LORD God." (Ezekiel 18: 7, 9)

"Honour thy father and thy mother: that thy days may be long upon the land which the LORD thy God giveth thee." (Exodus 20: 12)

"*Be* kindly affectioned one to another with brotherly love; in honour preferring one another." (Romans 12: 10)

Reflection(s): "Let it go!" Let nothing and no one get in the way of your march toward greater success, and always remain goal directed and focused on "winning the game". Make sure all the "dots connect" in a rational manner and avoid blockages of progress by others or yourself. In stressful, tense, and emotional situations, time to practice WWWST concepts by using your head, not your mouth until you calm down. Practice: "Let it go!"

Every person at birth starts life with a "good name" and excellent character standing. Such status may be maintained throughout childhood and adulthood or diminished, by choice. To maintain such positive status is simply a matter of doing the right things for the right reasons, not some of the time but all the time. One's honor is defined and enjoyed by self-actions, whether appreciated or not appreciated by others. It is left open to compliments or criticism, but always better to behave with honor and integrity. The idea of speaking and acting honorably is one of the most important choices a person can make, and it can be achieved 100% of the time.

Honor is important in terms of self-reflection and outward appearance. In history those who have been revered for being honorable have consistently demonstrated certain qualities, such as:

- Caring for others and for causes bigger than themselves.
- Joy in seeking to help others.
- Honesty.
- Trustworthiness.
- Understanding and an appreciation for loyalty.
- Comfort in showing love for self and others.
- Holding onto your principles and demonstrating honor even when pressured to behave otherwise -- "when they go low, we go high" mentality.

There are far more people in the world who live lives of honor than those who do not. People of honor do not have to announce or define their position. Yet, no one is perfect, and it is possible for a person to take actions on one day which are honorable and on other days to take actions which are not. It should not matter whether another person is watching. People of honor do the right thing whether they are being observed by other people.

There are some common terms that clearly define the difference between honorable and dishonorable conduct. For example, honorable people do not cheat; they do not steal; they do not violate the principles of teamwork and act as though they are part of one group and yet take actions of betrayal against the group for their own personal benefit. They take the time to help others any chance they get and are willing to put the greater good in service above themselves. Honorable people are loyal to family, co-workers, teammates, and others. Honorable people are honest, period -- not just some of the time but all the time! And they mind their own business and do not "mess with other people" for spite or otherwise; they leave other people alone. People of honor know and understand to tell the truth and do the right thing even when doing so at the time may be of some disadvantage to them, personally.

Character traits of honorable people are provided below; some are repeated above for emphasis. Think of how you and others you know demonstrate the character traits which follow:

- Fair.
- Credible.
- Concerned about other people and willing to show it.
- Positive in relating to others.
- Honest.
- Full of integrity.
- Loyal.
- Sensitive, no bullying or teasing of others.
- Not discriminatory based upon income levels, class, or race.
- Trustworthy.

I was proud of and thankful for my childhood growth environment for being surrounded by my family, friends, teachers, and church worshippers who were honorable people. The same goes for my adult life. It is a choice I decided to make long ago to surround myself with people of great honor and integrity. At any hint of people being dishonorable, I have always quickly moved away from those people. You can usually tell the difference within minutes, whether people are of honor or not.

I have learned that most people are honorable, hardworking and intend to do good things. We do more toward ensuring a peaceful and friendly environment by showing an attitude of grace and encouragement over discouragement. It is more rewarding for all concerned to believe things can change for the better; I have kept the faith and believe in things hoped for and the evidence of things not yet seen. Practice!

Reader - Think; Share; Reflect: _____

_____

_____

8. Honesty - Tell the truth and think, act, and live truthfully in all communications and transactions. Honesty is important whether related to the commission or omission of actions or comments in pursuance of the truth. Even in cases where the truth is not apparent or may be hidden from open view or misunderstood, the best approach is to "fill in the blanks" for accuracy rather than to allow misperceptions or lack of access to truth to prevail. Practice!

> *Alignment with Bible Passages:*

"*He that* speaketh truth sheweth forth righteousness: but a false witness deceit." (Proverbs 12:17)

"Lying lips *are* abomination to the LORD: but they that deal truly *are* his delight." (Proverbs 12:22)

"And ye shall know the truth, and the truth shall make you free." (John 8: 32)

"For he that will love life, and see good days, let him refrain his tongue from evil, and his lips that they speak no guile: let him eschew evil, and do good; let him seek peace, and ensue it." (1 Peter 3: 10-11)

"But now ye also put off all these; anger, wrath, malice, blasphemy, filthy communication out of your mouth. Lie not one to another, seeing that ye have put off the old man with his deeds; And have put on the new *man*, which is renewed in knowledge after the image of him that created him." (Colossians 3: 8-10)

"Thou shalt not bear false witness against thy neighbour." (Exodus 20: 16)

"For the wrath of God is revealed from heaven against all ungodliness and unrighteousness of men, who hold truth in unrighteousness." (Romans 1: 18)

"But speak thou the things which become sound doctrine: . . . In all things shewing thyself a pattern of good works: in doctrine *shewing* uncorruptness, gravity, sincerity, Sound speech, that cannot be condemned; that he is of the contrary part may be ashamed, having no evil thing to say of you." (Titus 2: 1, 7-8)

"Let no corrupt communication proceed out of your mouth, but that which is good to the use of edifying, that it may minister grace unto the hearers." (Ephesians 4: 29)

"If any man among you seem to be religious, and bridleth not his tongue, but deceiveth his own heart, this man's religion *is* vain." (James 1: 26)

Reflection(s): "Let it go!" Let nothing and no one get in the way of your march toward greater success, and always remain goal directed and focused on "winning the game". Make sure all the "dots connect" in a rational manner and avoid blockages of progress by others or yourself. In stressful, tense, and emotional situations, time to practice WWWST concepts by using your head, not your mouth until you calm down. Practice: "Let it go!"

It is important to tell the truth, all the time, even when not convenient and when the consequences that follow may feel quite uncomfortable. Everyone prefers to spend time with honest people -- friends or foes. Once a person is exposed as dishonest or lacking in his or her tendencies to be truthful, others will listen differently and cautiously, with hesitation in determining whether to believe what is being communicated. Better to just tell the truth, each time!

Note the following true story about honesty. Carolyn and I traveled through an unfamiliar city late one night in the state of Louisiana, and we were hungry. We stopped at the only fast-food restaurant in sight. We bought hamburgers and drinks for a total cost of $16.49. My wife gave the cashier a $20.00 bill, expecting $3.51 in change. The cashier mistakenly gave back $16.49, and my wife attempted to explain that this was the incorrect amount. Thinking that we were lodging a complaint, the cashier did not understand why there was a problem. We showed her the money she had given us, making her realize that she had returned to us the cost of the meal instead of the change amount. Upon understanding her mistake, she thanked us for being honest and said that it had been a long night and she was tired.

By returning the money to the cashier my wife demonstrated honesty and doing the right thing. She made a choice regarding not profiting from someone else's mistake. How would you have handled the situation? Why?

Think about your own stories where you or another person exhibited an honest response or reaction in a situation. Consider, for example, being approached by a person of some authority: a parent, schoolteacher or school administrator, police officer, manager of a store or other authority figure. You are thought to have observed a violation of the rules or law, perhaps even an accidental mishap. If approached to serve as a witness to report on what you have observed, what are your thoughts and attitude about how best to approach such a situation? It is just as much an act of dishonesty to hold onto the truth by saying nothing as it is to directly make a dishonest statement.

I was privileged to serve as the first head basketball coach of the current L. C. Anderson High School in Austin, Texas. I can recall vividly a situation where a mistake was made by a referee during a game against the Austin High School team in awarding the ball to the opposing team that should have been awarded to our team. The opposing coach acknowledged the mistake and informed the referee of the mistake simultaneously as our team coaches, players and fans complained. The referee corrected the mistake and awarded the ball to our team but only after the coach of the opposing team spoke. This is a fine demonstration of honesty by the coach, even with the awareness that such honesty would not be beneficial to his team. We won the game, but the opposing coach won a lot of respect for being honest.

My wife, Carolyn, has shared the story of how she returned $4.00 to the cashier of a large grocery store that she had found lying on the ground in the parking lot, while shopping with two of our three children. She explained to them and the cashier that honesty is the best practice. She was aware that the chances were not good that the person who lost the money would return to claim it and prove it belonged to them, and she believed it to be possible that the clerk may pocket the money for themselves. Her conscience was clear that she had done the right thing. I can recall being fortunate in a couple of similar circumstances and not so fortunate in another. In the case of not being so fortunate, I remember the situation where I was shopping at a store and upon presenting the cashier with a large bill, she returned to me the change from the purchase, and I placed it in my front right pocket, same pocket as I had placed my automobile keys. When I arrived at my vehicle and reached into my pocket to retrieve the keys, the money unknowingly fell out of my pocket. I left the parking lot and remembered moments later that I had placed the money in my pants pocket. I returned to check to see if the money may still be there where I must have dropped it; it was not. I checked with the store management, but no luck in the money being turned in to them -- lesson learned. On a more positive side and outcomes, I recall a couple of times where I dropped my wallet in the rest room, once at a service station in Texas and the other time at the airport in Los Angeles, California. In both cases the wallet was returned to me. With respect to the service station situation, the person who found the wallet ran into the parking lot to catch me before leaving. I was so proud and thankful that I offered a reward and later sent a congratulatory letter to management to express appreciation about the employee who had returned the wallet to me. In the case of the airport scenario, I touched the back of my pants and noticed the wallet was not in my pocket after leaving the rest room. The cleaner who had picked up the wallet later returned it to me.

What would you have done in finding money in the parking lot or rest room that did not belong to you? Practice! Honesty is always the best policy. The way to enrich yourself should not come resulting from the misery of another person but through hard work and doing the right things in the right way at the right time, including being honest all the time. Practice!

Reader - Think; Share; Reflect: _____

_____

_____

9. Listening - To listen is a major component in communication and is as important as speaking. There is a major difference in hearing and listening. Hearing simply perceives the sounds, while listening requires hearing the sounds and applying what is heard to a sense of meaning and determining an appropriate response, if any. Hearing is a natural function of the body in acknowledgement of sound; listening requires thinking and action. Practice!

➤ *Alignment with Bible Passages:*

"Wherefore, my beloved brethren, let every man be swift to hear, slow to speak, slow to wrath." (James 1:19)

"He *is* in the way of life that keepeth instruction: but he that refuseth reproof erreth." (Proverbs 10:17)

"The way of a fool *is* right in his own eyes: but he that hearkeneth unto counsel *is* wise." (Proverbs 12: 15)

"He that answereth a matter before he heareth it, it *is* folly and shame unto him." (Proverbs 18: 13)

"Therefore whatsoever ye have spoken in darkness shall be heard in the light; and that which ye have spoken in the ear in closets shall be proclaimed upon the housetops." (Luke 12: 3)

"Therefore whosoever heareth these sayings of mine, and doeth them, I will liken him unto a wise man, which built his house upon a rock: And the rain descended, and the floods came, and the winds blew, and beat upon that house; and it fell not: for it was founded upon a rock. And every one that heareth these sayings of mine, and doeth them not, shall be likened unto a foolish man, which built his house upon the sand: And the rain descended, and the floods came, and the winds blew, and beat upon that house; and it fell: and great was the fall of it." (Matthew 7: 24-27)

"But be ye doers of the word, and not hearers only, deceiving your own selves." (James 1: 22)

"But they obeyed not, neither inclined their ear, but made their neck stiff, that they might not hear, nor receive instruction." (Jeremiah 17: 23)

"Call unto me, and I will answer thee, and shew thee great and mighty things, which thou knowest not." (Jeremiah 33: 3)

"Moreover if thy brother shall trespass against thee, go and tell him his fault between thee and him alone: if he shall hear thee, thou hast gained thy brother." (Matthew 18: 15)

Reflection(s): "Let it go!" Let nothing and no one get in the way of your march toward greater success, and always remain goal directed and focused on "winning the game". Make sure all the "dots connect" in a rational manner and avoid blockages of progress by others or yourself. In stressful, tense, and emotional situations, time to practice WWWST concepts by using your head, not your mouth until you calm down. Practice: "Let it go!"

To listen requires thinking and action and not passive hearing of sounds. That is, listening requires making a deliberate attempt to process what is heard and analyzing it for meaning and determination of an appropriate response that is required or expected. It is, therefore, possible for a person to decide to actively not listen, even though the spoken words are heard. Listening requires blocking out of the mind or line of thinking any sounds which may distract from the meaning or intended purpose of the message being delivered.

In my many years of professional life, I have participated in numerous meetings and programs, some as a guest, others requiring attendance as an employee, and some as the host or supervisor -- calling for others to attend. I have worked at and been determined not to allow myself to be distracted during meetings, whether the topic of discussion or discussant was exciting or boring or somewhere in between. I am clear that it is important to listen to every word, whether the conversation is on a personal or professional level -- one or two words in meaning can make a major difference. I believe that much of the knowledge which I have attained has been the result of active listening. Actively listening means to practice the WAPP component, "what to say, when to say it, and when to stop talking". Is it always easy? No, so practice, practice, practice as other winners always do.

Any success I have enjoyed is related to and the result of my listening to others. For example, I listened to my mother, father, teachers, and pastor about the importance of staying in school and succeeding in school from elementary school through earning the doctorate at The University of Texas at Austin. I listened when my father repeated to me over and over this quote: "You can take a horse to water, but you cannot make him drink". It was a reminder to "let it go" and not push others into something they are not committed to doing. I listened to my high school basketball coaches who told me that I could succeed in college in basketball, prior to my signing a college letter of intent to attend Southwest Texas State University (current name - Texas State University) as the first African American athlete. I listened to parents, friends and teachers who instructed classmates and me never to quit something which you enjoy and may bring meaning into your life, saying routinely, "If you believe it, you can achieve it," and "If at first you don't succeed, try, try again." I have also listened to my wife and children and enjoyed conversations about the importance of family love and appreciation. Additionally, I listened to several physicians about the importance of living a healthy lifestyle and making important choices that enhance quality of life. Finally, I listened to and benefited from the advice of family, friends, and mentors within and across several groups not to engage in physical fights and not to do drugs. These individuals also helped me gain appreciation for and understanding of the importance of getting along with everyone and making it a routine practice to reach out to help others.

How many times have you observed or been part of a conversation where people talked at or toward each other but one or more of the participants did not listen -- heard the words but did not listen? Such communication is not helpful in general life conversations or sports teams' activities. Think about it. You are in the huddle of a football or basketball game or practice and a play is called, and one or more fail to listen, and they get the wrong understanding of which play is called. The play cannot work as successfully as it would have if everyone operated based upon what was expected. The play is going to the right and one or more players go to the left would not be a good outcome coming out of the huddle. A doctor tells the patient to take one pill every 8 hours to lead toward healing an ailment, and the patient who is not listening thinks he or she hears take one pill every hour for 8 hours would not lead to correction of the medical problem and could result in additional pain and suffering. A student in any school classroom half-listens to the teacher on a regular basis and test time wonders why he or she is not well-prepared to take the test. It is not an overstatement to say that the skills for effective listening are as important as those skills necessary for being an effective speaker. Effective listening is a necessity for success in sports and life.

The idea of developing and maintaining effective listening skills takes continuous practice and laser focus. In fact, you cannot be almost an effective listener, while noting that you listen much or some of the time; that is not a sign of being effective. It is also not appropriate in communication to block out those things over which you may not be interested and demonstrate a pattern of being a part-time listener. Practice!

Reader - Think; Share; Reflect: _____

_____

_____

10. Love (give and seek over hatred) - To love and be loved are equally important and a significant part of enjoying a successful lifestyle. Love, in a real sense, is connected within and across every emotion, thought and action; although, you cannot see it and touch it. It is always there. Each one of us wants to be loved and appreciated, and each one of us has the innate ability to give and receive love. There is no room or good time in a "high

quality" lifestyle for hatred, either to spread, devote time to it in thoughts or actions, or to experience it. Practice!

➢ *Alignment with Bible Passages:*

"A new commandment I give unto you, That ye love one another; as I have loved you, that ye also love one another. By this shall all *men* know that ye are my disciples, if ye have love one to another." (John 13: 34-35)

"But the fruit of the Spirit is love, joy, peace, long-suffering, gentleness, goodness, faith, Meekness, temperance: against such there is no law." (Galatians 5:22-23)

"And the second (commandment) *is* like, *namely* this, Thou shalt love thy neighbour as thyself. There is none other commandment greater than these." (Mark 12: 31)

"Ye have heard that it hath been said, Thou shalt love thy neighbour, and hate thine enemy. But I say unto you, Love your enemies, bless them that curse you, do good to them that hate you, and pray for them which despitefully use you, and persecute you; That ye may be the children of your Father which is in heaven: for he maketh his sun to rise on the evil and on the good, and sendeth rain on the just and on the unjust. For if ye love them which love you, what reward have ye? do not even the publicans the same? And if ye salute your brethren only, what do ye more *than others*? do not even the publicans so? Be ye therefore perfect, even as your Father which is in heaven is perfect." (Matthew 5: 43-48)

"*Let* love be without dissimulation. Abhor that which is evil; cleave to that which is good. *Be* kindly affectioned one to another with brotherly love; in honour preferring one another . . . Bless them which persecute you: bless, and curse not. Rejoice with them that do rejoice, and weep with them that weep . . . Recompense to no man evil for evil. Provide things honest in the sight of all men. If it be possible, as much as lieth in you, live peaceably with all men . . . Therefore if thine enemy hunger, feed him; if he thirst, give him drink: for in so doing thou shalt heap coals of fire on his head. Be not overcome of evil, but overcome evil with good." (Romans 12: 9-10; 14-15; 17-18; 20-21)

"Owe no man any thing, but to love one another: for he that loveth another hath fulfilled the law. For this, Thou shalt not commit adultery, Thou shalt not kill, Thou shalt not steal, Thou shalt not bear false witness, Thou shalt not covet; and if *there be* any other commandment, it is briefly comprehended in this saying, namely, Thou shalt love thy neighbour as thyself." (Romans 13: 8-10)

"And let us consider one another to provoke unto love and to good works." (Hebrews 10:24)

"The mouth of a righteous *man is* a well of life: but violence covereth the mouth of the wicked. Hatred stirreth up strifes: but love covereth all sins." (Proverbs 10: 11-12)

"Charity suffereth long, *and* is kind; charity envieth not; charity vaunteth not itself, is not puffed up, Doth not behave itself unseemly, seeketh not her own, is not easily provoked, thinketh no evil; Rejoiceth not in iniquity, but rejoiceth in the truth; Beareth all things, believeth all things, hopeth all things, endureth all things . . . And now abideth faith, hope, charity, these three; but the greatest of these *is* charity." (1 Corinthians 13: 4-7; 13)

"To every *thing there is* a season, and a time to every purpose under the heaven. . . A time to love, and a time to hate; a time of war, and a time of peace. (Ecclesiastes 3: 1; 8)

Reflection(s): "Let it go!" Let nothing and no one get in the way of your march toward greater success, and always remain goal directed and

45

focused on "winning the game". Make sure all the "dots connect" in a rational manner and avoid blockages of progress by others or yourself. In stressful, tense, and emotional situations, time to practice WWWST concepts by using your head, not your mouth until you calm down. Practice: "Let it go!"

I have been fortunate to enjoy true love within and across family, high school and college school classmates, neighbors, church members, and co-workers. Each experience has been grounded in shared, two-way mutual understandings and support. In growing up the love umbrella included my birth family and other relatives: mother and father, sisters and brothers, grandparents, uncles and aunts, and cousins. The love has been strong and unconditional, mutual, and unwavering in the way it has been shared.

The fortune of enjoying true love has continued and grown with the marriage of my wife, Carolyn, and birth, growth, and development of our son and two daughters: Berlin Lee Brown, Mary Katherine (Brown) Ruegg and Reesha Johnette (Brown) Edwards and granddaughter, Abigail Sage Ruegg. Each day has been filled with love and affection and support throughout our time together. The in-laws, through marriage, have also been welcoming, supportive and strong in their love and encouragement. One proud example of the love we have all shared is our advocacy for and appreciation of diversity. So, it is no surprise that our youngest daughter attended her high school senior class prom in the company of a diverse group of other students -- via limousine, which our family proudly sponsored. And, no surprise that our family includes bi-racial marriages, and the union of these families together has been very friendly and refreshingly positive.

I can recall many, many examples of expressions of love throughout my life. One example is the time when I left home for college, and my father took what he said was his last money savings he was keeping for dental care and gave it to me for college start-up supplies and well-being. We were economically challenged and, yet, not hungry or experiencing suffering conditions. As a family we always had what we needed, and we counted upon each other for support. My mother was always strong in showing encouragement and unconditional love, even when correcting my brothers, sisters, and me. I sometimes wondered during childhood where she got the energy from, as she would be up early in the morning and late in the evening taking care of the children. She was constantly busy with church and community endeavors in reaching out to help others. She modeled that which she preached, "Take time to help somebody every day". She routinely questioned me and my siblings about what we had done to assist other people and to explain how. She loved her community and church friends and family and showed it up to the date of her death. My father constantly demonstrated love for the family as well. He, too, was always busy working on the job and after work building and refining things at home during my childhood and up to the time of his death. The house lawn was always well-manicured, and flowers and vegetables that he had planted were plentiful. He built a gazebo in our back yard and garage and added a room onto the back of the house, so that we would have more space for our family consisting of him, my mother and six children. Both of my parents were strict about our being successful in school. They understood that the best route for their children to enjoy happiness and well-being as adults was through gaining an excellent education. Carolyn's parents showed the same love and support for Carolyn, her brothers, and sister, according to stories she has shared and my own observations before her parents died. It should be no surprise that Carolyn and I have done our best to show the same love, support, and attention toward our son and two daughters (and granddaughter) throughout their childhood years and to date.

The family reunions on my mother's side of the family occurred routinely, at least once per year and more frequently some years during my childhood and young adult years, primarily in Bryan, Texas, my mother's birthplace. Such gatherings included my mother's parents, sisters and brother and their spouses and my brothers, sisters, and cousins. There was always a lot of food and friendly conversation. Although, there were occasions when it was difficult to pass the test of knowing the name of certain relatives -- that is, responding to the question: "Do you know who I am", time after time, year after year. The reunions would also occur at my home in Austin and, occasionally, in Houston. The love, joy, and caring were always overflowing and genuine. My father did not often travel out of town, so he would not attend except when the reunions were held at our house. I do not recall such reunions with my father's side of the family. Carolyn's family on her father's side also enjoyed reunions during her developing years up to and including several years after our wedding. The family would gather primarily at her home in Paris, Texas and would include family members from West Texas and the state of Oklahoma; occasions which were always full of love and caring for one another. I regret that we have not continued such traditions in recent years. Yet, the families within and across my family and Carolyn's were joined for two special occasions, the wedding ceremonies of our daughters, Mary and Reesha. For those two joyous occasions relatives and friends from Austin, Dallas, Paris, Houston, and Port Arthur in Texas and from the states of Minnesota, Oregon, Georgia, and Arizona attended. Our family also enjoyed the pleasure of celebrating together in love and joy at the high school and college graduation ceremonies of Berlin, Mary and Reesha. We had a little more excitement than we had counted upon following Reesha's graduation from The University of West Georgia, as the sirens warning of a tornado blasted in the air just as we were leaving the ceremony. Tornadoes did ravage the area of Metro-Atlanta, Georgia but we were all fortunate to avoid injury.

The experiences at Texas State University and The University of Texas were positive from start to finish, throughout my higher education training experiences, whereupon as students we routinely demonstrated love for one another. In both schools I was one of a few African American students in my college programs and classes. The same love and joy held true for my work experiences and faith-based involvement, as the high regard, support and love have been more prevalent than not in interactions among colleagues. I have been fortunate to heed the advice I was given and swift to share with the youth and others: "hang around those people who will take you up in life" and not around those who will take you down with them. In heeding such advice, I have been fortunate to enjoy success, joy, and loving environments in all phases of life. I happen to believe there is good in each person, and better to look for it than to assume otherwise. At the start as a baby every person begins with the potential to become a loving and pleasant child and adult.

Everyone needs and wants to be loved and appreciated. Yet not all will admit it, and far too many do not show love in return. I am most fortunate and proud of being surrounded by such a loving family. Our family is also proudly diverse by race and backgrounds. And our family has routinely been advocates for celebrating diversity and looking at different races and cultures as opportunities to share in experiences and rich dialogue.

How often do you use the word or think about love in an expression of care, concern, and appreciation for another person? Once or twice a month? Once or twice a week? Every day? Men are often more reluctant than women to verbally express their thoughts and feelings in such direct terms -- should not be that way, but that is the reality. Love is something that every person needs, appreciates and is capable of sharing. Love is so valuable that everyone is encouraged to enjoy it, look for opportunities to spread it widely in communication among others and feel comfortable in expressing it in words and actions.

One of the common themes in songs and literature is love. It is so common, at least partly, because it is a strong reminder of the importance of affection, admiration, and well-being which everyone wants and needs to experience and share. Love is associated with happiness, joy, comfort, passion, care and concern, commitment, and a range of emotions. I am a strong arts advocate, including appreciation for and enjoyment of music. For example, I enjoy attending concerts featuring my favorite artists, and routinely listening to popular love songs, such as those listed below and many more (emphasizing enjoyment listening to the bands and singers):

- "Endless Love", featuring Lionel Richie and Diana Ross – youtube.com (1981)
- "Greatest Love of All", featuring Whitney Houston- youtube. com (2010- originally released – 1985);
- "I Will Always Love You", featuring Whitney Houston – youtube.com (1994);
- "Stone in Love With You", featuring The Stylistics – youtube. com (1972);
- "That's What Friends are for", featuring Dionne & Friends (including Dionne Warwick,

Elton Jon, Gladys Knight, and Stevie Wonder) – youtube.com (1985).
Practice! Finish this sentence routinely for a smile each day on the meaning of love to you - - Love is . . .

Reader - Think; Share; Reflect: _____

_____

_____

11. Loyalty - Loyalty is an important factor for achieving a common goal. Once the members of the group are identified and the group norms are established, there is an expectation of loyalty or agreement with all members of the team or group. Membership will change over time, with new members added and others leaving the group. Once norms are clear and established and there is a goal in mind for winning or high achievement, everyone must believe in and practice the concept of counting on other members of the group and being counted upon, as a loyal or committed member of the group. Practice!

➤ *Alignment with Bible Passages*:

"A friend loveth at all times, and a brother is born for adversity. A man void of understanding striketh hands, *and* becometh surety in the presence of his friend." (Proverbs 17: 17-18)

"A man *that hath* friends must shew himself friendly: and there is a friend *that* sticketh closer than a brother." (Proverbs 18: 24)

"Most men will proclaim every one his own goodness: but a faithful man who can find?" (Proverbs 20: 6)

"He that followeth after righteousness and mercy findeth life, righteousness and honour." (Proverbs 21: 21)

"Thine own friend, and thy father's friend, forsake not; neither go into thy brother's house in the day of thy calamity: *for* better *is* a neighbour *that is* near than a brother far off." (Proverbs 27: 10)

"Greater love hath no man than this, that a man lay down his life for his friends." (John 15:13)

"They went out from us, but they were not of us; for if they had been of us, they would *no doubt* have continued with us: but *they went out*, that they might be made manifest that they were not all of us." (1 John 2: 19)

"Help, LORD; for the godly man ceaseth; for the faithful fail from among the children of men. They speak vanity every one with his neighbour: *with* flattering lips *and* with a double heart do they speak." (Psalm 12: 1-2)

"Let the husband render unto the wife due benevolence: and likewise also the wife unto the husband. The wife hath not power of her own body, but the husband: and likewise also the husband hath not power of his own body, but the wife." (1 Corinthians 7: 3-4)

"*Be* kindly affectioned one to another with brotherly love; in honour preferring one another." (Romans 12: 10)

Reflection(s): "Let it go!" Let nothing and no one get in the way of your march toward greater success, and always remain goal directed and focused on "winning the game". Make sure all the "dots connect" in a rational manner and avoid blockages of progress by others or yourself. In stressful, tense, and emotional situations, time to practice WWWST concepts by using your head, not your mouth until you calm down. Practice: "Let it go!"

Loyalty is a two-way proposition -- you to the team or organization and the team or organization to you. True loyalty is earned on both sides and entails promises and agreements made and kept. Loyalty is not, and should not be, contingent upon nor a mechanism to stifle disagreements. Rather, it should be based upon commonly agreed upon terms, verbal and written, which express mutual benefits for the team or organization and individual. Mutual benefit means that neither the team nor organization acts or is involved in activities that may be harmful or disruptive. Loyalty is earned and not easily broken and, yet, when lost it is difficult to be renewed.

There are clear advantages in the "team" concept, "all for one and one for all" mentality. I have enjoyed actively practicing the "team" approach as early as childhood and through the "world of work" in employment. Indeed, when the team or organization has a "weak link" in the group, any adverse comments or actions can result in a negative effect and, even, disastrous consequences for all concerned. Consider, for example, the effect of disloyalty and lack of dedication and commitment in an organization such as a circus trapeze act, where one mistake in technique may result in tragedy. Practice leads toward perfection, and not practicing may lead to disaster. And consider a basketball team where a person refuses to practice free throws and that person on the team is faced with an opportunity to win the game with a few seconds left on the clock. Again, practicing leads toward perfection.

I have been most fortunate to participate on athletic teams in high school and college and in employment in associating myself with persons with a strong sense of what it means to be loyal. For example, when managers at segregated hotels and restaurants refused service to the Texas State University basketball team and fans at games yelled racial slurs because of my presence, the coaches and other players never wavered in their support for me. The team was loyal and supportive in each situation we encountered.

If a person is unhappy or disgruntled with the team or organization, it is important to address the matter through established procedures and protocols. Also, never, ever give up when you know you are right, and the facts are on your side and the team or organization is better served by your pursuit of the decision you are seeking.

A person who demonstrates loyalty toward another person, organization or team is also demonstrating traits of teamwork and trustworthiness at the same time -- that is -- three WAPP components in one action. In fact, if either of these components is missing, there is a question whether true loyalty is accomplished. Yet it is important to acknowledge that what and to whom you are showing loyalty to is for the right reasons and of high integrity and high moral character. Make sure your loyalty is not misplaced. Practice!

Reader - Think; Share; Reflect: _____

_____

_____

12. Protect property (of self and others and not steal) - It is not complicated. There is no good reason to steal or even think about it. Besides being the wrong thing to do by law and violation in morality, stealing is hurtful to both self and others. It does not matter that no one is around to see you steal; it is just as wrong. At the same time, it is important to plan for and take actions to protect one's own property. Take steps even as simple as keeping keys or wallet in the same, exact place while traveling or sleeping or locking the door behind you for safety and protection of property. Think, plan, practice!

> ➢ *Alignment with Bible Passages*:

"Thou shalt not steal." (Exodus: 20: 15)

"Let him that stole steal no more: but rather let him labour, working with *his* hands the thing which is good, that he may have to give to him that needeth." (Ephesians 4: 28)

"Thou therefore which teachest another, teachest thou not thyself? thou that preachest a man should not steal, dost thou steal? (Romans 2: 21)

"Lay not up for yourselves treasures upon earth, where moth and rust doth corrupt, and where thieves break through and steal: But lay up for yourselves treasures in heaven, where neither moth nor rust doth corrupt, and where thieves do not break through nor steal: For where your treasure is, there will your heart be also." (Matthew 6:19-21)

"My son, if sinners entice thee, consent thou not. If they say, Come with us, let us lay wait for blood, let us lurk privily for the innocent without cause: Let us swallow them up alive as the grave; and whole, as those that go down into the pit: We shall find all precious substance, we shall fill our houses with spoil: Cast in thy lot among us; let us all have one purse: My son, walk not thou in the way with them; refrain thy foot from their path." (Proverbs 1: 10-15)

"And my people shall dwell in a peaceable habitation, and in sure dwellings, and in quiet resting places." (Isaiah 32: 18)

"Because thou hast made the LORD, *which is* my refuge, *even* the most high, thy habitation; There shall no evil befall thee, neither shall any plague come nigh thy dwelling. For he shall give his angels charge over thee, to keep thee in all thy ways." (Psalm 91: 9-11)

"When a strong man armed keepeth his palace, his goods are in peace." (Luke 11: 21)

"Again, when I say unto the wicked, Thou shalt surely die; if he turn from his sin, and do that which is lawful and right; *If* the wicked restore the pledge, give again that he had robbed, walk in the statutes of life, without committing iniquity; he shall surely live, he shall not die . . . When the righteous turneth from his righteousness, and committeth iniquity, he shall even die thereby. But if the wicked turn from his wickedness, and do that which is lawful and right, he shall live thereby." (Ezekiel 33: 14-15; 18-19)

"Verily I say unto you, Whosoever shall not receive the kingdom of God as a little child shall in no wise enter therein. And a certain ruler asked him, saying, Good Master, what shall I do to inherit eternal life? And Jesus said unto him, Why callest thou me good? none *is* good, save one, *that is,* God. Thou knowest the commandments, Do not commit adultery, Do not kill, Do not steal, Do not bear false witness, Honour thy father and thy mother." (Luke 18: 17-20)

Reflection(s): "Let it go!" Let nothing and no one get in the way of your march toward greater success, and always remain goal directed and focused on "winning the game". Make sure all the "dots connect" in a rational manner and avoid blockages of progress by others or yourself. In stressful, tense, and emotional situations, time to practice WWWST concepts by using your head, not your mouth until you calm down. Practice: "Let it go!"

I was excited upon earning a "letter jacket" from my high school in recognition of success in athletics, following the season of my junior year at the school. About a year later I was not so pleased when the jacket was stolen while friends and I were enjoying time together at the local neighborhood area elementary school. Neither my friends nor I observed the person stealing the jacket. It was out of sight for only a few moments, but I should have been more careful to wear the jacket or maintain sight of it to avoid my property being stolen. The jacket was taken by one of my former classmates and maintained and worn for over 20 years before the person decided to return it through a relative who remained in Austin. The former classmate expressed being overcome by feelings of guilt and decided the way to correct the wrong action was to return the jacket to me through the relative. My family member simply thanked the person for returning the jacket; although, it had an appearance of being old and worn. I was proud of myself and family for demonstrating the ability to "let it go" and move on. I never attempted to identify the person who committed the act of taking the jacket which did not belong to him. I was simply pleased that the jacket was returned to me.

Hurricane Harvey, which occurred during the last few days of August and the start of September 2017, was a true test on the ability to "let it go". The storm drenched Southeast Texas with rain for several days, totaling more measurable inches of rain than over hundreds of years. The storm was a "direct hit" over Port Arthur, Texas, the city in which Carolyn and I reside. Over 80 per cent of homes and businesses in the area were flooded, including our home. The worst day and night of the storm was August 29. The rain poured down all day and night and early the next morning. The storm's effect on us and our property was most challenging, and things got more serious as the storm sewer system broke down, resulting in flooding of homes and businesses throughout the city.

We made attempts to protect our home from flooding through what we thought were common sense actions, such as stacking towels and "throw rugs" at each house entrance -- front and back doors and garage door. We even made attempts to cover the bottom of tables and chairs with plastic bags to prevent water damage. Such actions were no match for "mother nature". Our efforts were no match for the water rising inside our house. By the end of the day, August 29, we observed that despite our intense efforts to protect our property, water began to seep through cracks in and around the doors, walls, and foundation of the house; we had lost our battle with the storm for sure at approximately 7:00 p.m. The carpet on the floors in our master and other bedrooms filled quickly with water at that point. The water in the garage rose quickly as well. Our pet Chihuahua showed signs of panic -- like the panic that he must have observed in the faces of Carolyn and me.

The time had come to gather the essentials and move to the upstairs area of the house. Fortunately, we had that as an option. The time had come to "let it go" for now and focus on survival and deal with the property interests later. The neighbors next door and we communicated several times throughout the night. For example, we talked about issues such as the need to ensure the electrical breakers were turned off as soon as possible. The house construction contractor -- who lives in the same neighborhood -- alerted us to be sure that to prevent electrical shock, we should wear rubber boots or some type of foot covering in the house prior to attempting to turn off the breakers.

If one were to raise the questions of how serious the situation was and why we and others did not leave prior to the flooding, the answers may be easily given: a. How serious? The flooding was so bad we had to depart in a boat; b. Why not leave earlier? The water rose very quickly, and conditions worsened beyond what was anticipated due to the amount of rain, and the sewage drainage system broke down in the middle of the storm. Roads and highways were flooded and closed for many miles, leaving automobiles inoperable. Hotels were flooded as well. The Civic Center which was opened as a local shelter was also flooded to the point that those who sought shelter there were required to sit in the bleachers.

We were fortunate that our next-door neighbor contacted friends who own a boat and were most generous with their time and efforts to lift several neighbors and my wife and me out of harm's way. The street flooding was so bad that the water sat in the streets a couple of weeks in some areas, making travel on those streets impassable. We were also fortunate to gain access to a local church shelter for an overnight stay, and we gained access to one of the few available hotel rooms for the following night. We remained in various local hotels for about four months, sponsored by the United States Government – Federal Emergency Management Agency (FEMA) for which we are eternally grateful. Such support came only after numerous phone calls and emails, however. FEMA also provided temporary shelter in the form of a trailer which was placed on our home property for several months, pending completion of repairs to our home. We were quite privileged to enjoy such an opportunity, which enabled us to be in a better position to protect our property and curtail our stint of living in hotels. We were more than ready to go home by this point. Regrettably, the management in some of the hotels implemented regulations that restricted room availability to cash paying customers only and, thereby, blocking access to those potential customers who were sponsored by FEMA. Such a practice wreaked of unfair housing discrimination intended to accept for housing only affluent customers, thereby, blocking access to many Southeast Texas residents. Carolyn and I were fortunate to avoid direct impact of such discriminatory practices.

The transition from the flood, staying in hotels and living in the trailer took over a year and a half before we were able to move back into our home. The work from "gutting" the house of carpet, walls, tile floors and furniture, followed by the required renovation work and replacement of appliances and furniture took a lot of patience and money. We were fortunate to have flood and windstorm insurance, for sure. Yet, by living in a somewhat rural area, the trustworthy contractors were limited in number. We kept the faith – in things hoped for and the evidence of things not yet seen.

If something you own is important to you, make sure you put the conditions in place to protect it. How about leaving your automobile or home unlocked late into the night after you have gone to bed? Is that the proper way to protect property? No, it is not. How about loaning something valuable to a person who has routinely demonstrated themselves to be unreliable in the past; not smart and not an example of protecting property sufficiently. More profoundly be careful about loaning anything of value to anyone who does not live in your house or apartment.

I am fond of the memories of several moments of my visit to Banjul, The Gambia, West Africa. One such moment was the observance of a visit to a shopping market which featured several products: clothes, shoes, household items, food, and more. The storekeepers were very friendly to us, to the point of leaving their stores to walk with us from store to store, leaving the management of the stores to neighboring store owners/operators -- apparently not burdened with the fear of someone stealing or tampering with their property. It appeared to be quite an honor system, although a risky practice. It was a fine example of "brother's keeper" and brotherly love and concern. That is not to say the city does not have instances of property theft, mischief, or crime, but the expectations were incredibly strong that their property was safe in their absence due to the neighboring store owners assisting their neighbors' property interests. Afterall, such high expectations should be so strong among us all, as there is no ambiguity in the laws of any nation or in biblical terms, you should never steal. Whether the category is "white collar" crime relative to thousands of dollars or local market stores where the cost of products may range from less than one dollar to hundreds or thousands of dollars, people should protect their property, but others should also not steal it. Practice!

Reader - Think; Share; Reflect: _____

_____

_____

13. Reading - Reading is basic to all other knowledge, and it is key to all learning and the "spine" which holds everything together. If you cannot read, everybody will know it. Also, there is no "victory" in being illiterate. When you speak, your speech is a clear and public indicator of your level of preparation and intelligence. Reading is a means to acquire more tools and information for excellent communication skills. A person who is a poor or reluctant reader shows his or her lack of preparation and obvious unwillingness to grow in the skill set required for a good fit in society. You have a choice whether to be viewed as intelligent or unintelligent and, like any other skill set, you must practice each day to improve. Practice!

➤ *Alignment with Bible Passages*:

"The fear of the LORD *is* the beginning of knowledge: *but* fools despise wisdom and instruction. My son, hear the instruction of thy father, and forsake not the law of thy mother. For they *shall* be an ornament of grace unto thy head, and chains about thy neck." (Proverbs 1: 7-9)

"Wisdom *is* the principal thing; *therefore* get wisdom: and with all thy getting get understanding." (Proverbs 4:7)

"Every wise woman buildeth her house: but the foolish plucketh it down with her hands . . . The wisdom of the prudent *is* to understand his way: but the folly of fools *is* deceit." (Proverbs 14: 1; 8)

"The heart of him that hath understanding seeketh knowledge: but the mouth of fools feedeth on foolishness." (Proverbs 15:14)

"The wise in heart shall be called prudent: and the sweetness of the lips increaseth learning. Understanding *is* a wellspring of life unto him that hath it: but the instruction of fools *is* folly. The heart of the wise teacheth his mouth, and addeth learning to his lips. Pleasant words *are as* an honeycomb, sweet to the soul, and health to the bones." (Proverbs 16: 21-24)

"Day unto day uttereth speech, and night unto night sheweth knowledge." (Psalm 19: 2)

"Teach me good judgment and knowledge: for I have believed thy commandments." (Psalm 119: 66)

"Therefore whosoever heareth these sayings of mine, and doeth them, I will liken him unto a wise man, which built his house upon a rock: And the rain descended, and the floods came, and the winds blew, and beat upon that house; and it fell not: for it was founded upon a rock. And everyone that heareth these sayings of mine, and doeth them not, shall be likened unto a foolish man, which built his house upon the sand: And the rain descended, and the floods came, and the winds blew, and beat upon that house; and it fell: and great was the fall of it." (Matthew 7: 24-27)

"For wisdom *is* a defence, *and* money is a defence: but the excellency of knowledge is, *that* wisdom giveth life to them that have it." (Ecclesiastes 7: 12)

"For whatsoever things were written aforetime were written for our learning, that we through patience and comfort of the scriptures might have hope." (Romans 15: 4)

Reflection(s): "Let it go"! Let nothing and no one get in the way of your march toward greater success, and always remain goal directed and focused on "winning the game". Make sure all the "dots connect" in a rational manner and avoid blockages of progress by others or yourself. In stressful, tense, and emotional situations, time to practice WWWST concepts by using your head, not your mouth until you calm down. Practice: "Let it go"!

Reading is especially important! Read; read; read and read even more -- never enough! Reading is one of the most important skill sets imaginable. It is so important because reading is a requirement for all aspects of intelligence, knowledge, and communication. It is a fact that when you read, you grow in knowledge and skills through practice.

I read each day and have done so for many, many years; the same goes for my wife, Carolyn. I was fortunate to enjoy the experience as a first and second grade student, with Mrs. Poole and Mrs. Harris, who, along with my parents and siblings, ensured that my classmates and I were taught how and encouraged to read. Other teachers beyond second grade also did an excellent job in assuring the conditions were favorable for student success in reading. We learned early in life how important reading is in leading toward a happy, high quality lifestyle, and my parents and educators were right. Our lessons were consistent in substance, and teachers insisted that students practice at home. The terms were not necessarily announced during my early years why we practiced various aspects of our learning how to read successfully. However, as I advanced educationally and professionally, the need to possess good reading skills became quite clear. In reviewing current research and practice, the approach utilized by my grade school teachers was primarily consistent and aligned with basic understandings on how best to teach children how to read, including the following:

- Building phonemic awareness or sound segmentation strategies.
- Learning phonics and decoding of words.
- Practicing reading fluency and automatic recognition of words in text.
- Practicing vocabulary skills and increasing vocabulary banks over time.
- Comprehension of text while reading.
- Expression through writing.
- Connecting reading and writing to complement each other in increasing overall literacy.
- Emphasizing spelling, more often when I was in school than currently is required; and
- Practicing handwriting skills, again, more during my years in school than currently is required.

Upon becoming an educator, I was truly clear about the importance of all teachers encouraging children to read frequently and with fluency and strong comprehension. During the time of my experience as sports coach: football, basketball, track, tennis and swimming at the middle school level, and football and basketball at the high school level, I encouraged our athletes to read. Texas now has state laws about student athletes being required to "pass" to "play" or performing successfully in classes to participate in sports. As a coach I implemented rules for passing to play long before the state-imposed legislation for participation. "No pass-No play" under my direction as a coach went beyond the low-level expectation of passing. My rule as high school coach was that team members should make "A" s and "B" s in classes or face consequences. We established a culture of excellence where we expected our athletes to succeed, and they agreed through their actions and reports of success.

As coach I took the time each grading period to highlight the results of our hard work for excellent achievement in academics. I also expected the athletes to stay out of trouble in school and beyond. And together we established a culture of excellence and championship behavior as the norm. We enjoyed victories in the classroom and in winning games on the basketball court. As high school basketball coach at the L.C. Anderson High School in Austin, our record for our best year of performance was 24 wins and six losses, including only one loss in district play. I was honored to be selected as the Coach of the Year for that season. In our final game that year, we lost a "nail-biter" to John H. Reagan High School of Austin during a bi-district playoff game at Gregory Gymnasium at The University of Texas at Austin. We played the game in a larger gymnasium than our ordinary high school site due to the anticipated size of the audience. I considered our players to be champions in the classroom and as competitive athletes. I routinely emphasized reading before, during, and after the school days.

In determining what to read as an adult, I make deliberate efforts to mix it up every day: magazines; newspapers -- at least two to three per day; internet surfing; fiction and non-fiction novels; Bible; and professional literature. I find it to be refreshing and fun to spend time writing every chance I get, which is most days. I am proud to be part of a family of readers: from my birth family, including mother and father; sisters and brothers, and, wife, Carolyn; and our son and two daughters and sons-in-law.

Do you know anyone who avoids reading? It is never too late for them to start, if so. A little encouragement can go a long way. Perhaps gifting to them for their reading enjoyment a book or articles on a topic they appear to spend time talking about or appear to show interest in. This approach is good for encouraging adults and, especially, important in communicating with youth.

What is your skill level in reading? I was so honored to be presented with a book by a local area state judge written by David W. Blight - Frederick Douglass: Prophet of Freedom. The story was enlightening and informative. It was also written at a college reading level. See below a few of the words I lifted from the book to check whether your reading level is on par for knowledge, understanding and recognition of each word? Again, these words were lifted from one book, only. Remember, practice matters!

SAMPLE WORD LIST - Definitions are found in the back of the book.

1.	Absolution	19. Fictive	37. Polemical
2.	Amalgamation	20. Homiletic	38. Precociousness
3.	Ambivalence	21. Implacable	39. Profligate
4.	Antebellum	22. Impudence	40. Prolific
5.	Assiduously	23. Impunity	41. Propitious
6.	Avarice	24. Indefatigable	42. Rapacity
7.	Beguiling	25. Ineffaceably	43. Rebuked
8.	Benighted	26. Intelligible	44. Regal
9.	Buoyant	27. Intemperance	45. Repartee
10.	Capacious	28. Loquacity	46. Reproach
11.	Cataclysm	29. Magnanimity	47. Revelatory
12.	Clamorous	30. Mellifluous	48. Salacious
13.	Conviviality	31. Mendacity	49. Stultifying
14.	Decadence	32. Non-Sequitur	50. Stupendous
15.	Disconsolate	33. Ostentatious	51. Suasion
16.	Egalitarianism	34. Pacifism	52. Tempestuous
17.	Enmity	35. Peripatetic	53. Ubiquitous
18.	Expostulated	36. Poignant	54. Virulently

Reader - Think; Share; Reflect: _____

_____

_____

14. Respect (self and others and mind your business) - You deserve to be respected and so does everyone else. Respect starts with self and how you think and act and is apparent in all you say and do. It is far better to demonstrate positive regard toward others than to leave interpretation of your intent to chance. It is also important to give and receive respectful gestures and non-verbal cues in communication with other people. When confronted with decisions on whether to get involved or not, better to mind your own business, especially if the issue is not of your direct concern. Stay out of it. Practice!

> *Alignment with Bible Passages:*

Golden Rule: "Therefore all things whatsoever ye would that men should do to you, do ye even so to them: for this is the law and the prophets." (Matthew 7: 12)

"*Let* love be without dissimulation. Abhor that which is evil; cleave to that which is good. *Be* kindy affectioned one to another with brotherly love; in honour preferring one another." (Romans 12: 9-10)

"*Let* nothing *be done* through strife or vainglory; but in lowliness of mind let each esteem other better than themselves." (Philippians 2:3)

"Honour all *men.* Love the brotherhood. Fear God. Honour the king." (1

Peter 2:17)

"Even as I please all *men* in all *things*, not seeking mine own profit, but the *profit* of many, that they may be saved." (1 Corinthians 10: 33)

"For we dare not make ourselves of the number, or compare ourselves with some that commend themselves: but they measuring themselves by themselves, and comparing themselves among themselves, are not wise." (2 Corinthians 10: 12)

"A new commandment I give unto you, That ye love one another; as I have loved you, that ye also love one another. By this shall all *men* know that ye are my disciples, if ye have love one to another." (John 13: 34-35)

"He that oppresseth the poor reproacheth *his* Maker: but he that honoureth him hath mercy on the poor . . . Whoso mocketh the poor reproacheth *his* Maker: *and* he that is glad at calamities shall not be unpunished." (Proverbs 14: 31; 17: 5)

"In all things *shewing* thyself a pattern of good works: in doctrine *shewing* uncorruptness, gravity, sincerity, Sound speech, that cannot be condemned; that he that is of the contrary part may be ashamed, having no evil thing to say of you . . . For the grace of God that bringeth salvation hath appeared to all men, Teaching us that, denying ungodliness and worldly lusts, we should live soberly, righteously, and godly, in this present world." (Titus 2: 7-8; 11-12)

"And we beseech you, brethren, to know them which labour among you, and are over you in the LORD, and admonish you; And to esteem them very highly in love for their work's sake. *And* be at peace among yourselves." (1 Thessalonians 5: 12-13)

Reflection(s): "Let it go!" Let nothing and no one get in the way of your march toward greater success, and always remain goal directed and focused on "winning the game". Make sure all the "dots connect" in a rational manner and avoid blockages of progress by others or yourself. In stressful, tense, and emotional situations, time to practice WWWST concepts by using your head, not your mouth until you calm down. Practice: "Let it go!"

The idea of respecting oneself and others goes beyond words and direct actions. It is also a reflection and demonstration of one's attitude as demonstrated in verbal and non-verbal communication. There is much that can be accomplished, and progress made in communication, if only we look beyond our personal ideas on what a person should look or act like. People, whether intentionally or unintentionally, decide or make attempts to control what others say and do. Respecting another person should not depend upon whether that person follows the same approach as others may wish or think appropriate. In thinking like a champion, we should all work at <u>leaving other people alone, except to be helpful</u> and looking for ways to understand and support each other instead of dictating or criticizing. And always, always respect yourself.

Among other measures of strength and maturity of people in business, sports and entertainment is the show of comfort in acknowledging and applauding someone else for excellence in performance -- especially when they perform better at some skill or project than themselves. It takes a confident person to admit someone else is better at something, even if just momentarily. On the other hand, it is "small" and overly competitive and petty to know it and not acknowledge it. If you consider the definition of average, it is not possible for everyone or everything to be above average. Rather than sulk or complain that someone is better than you at something, it is better to praise the good and strive to improve, moving toward the level of performance or skill set that you admire in someone else. Be excited for your colleagues when they accomplish something special and let them know it.

I was fortunate to grow up in an environment where the family members respected one another, and the same held true among my teachers and classmates, church members and neighborhood. The respect spanned within and across all aspects of my Emerson Street childhood environment. Did we have disagreements among these groups? Yes, but we made deliberate attempts to demonstrate respect throughout our communication opportunities, whether we agreed or not. We expressed ourselves by sharing thoughts on situations or issues but not about individuals. There was no abuse, insults, "put downs", or any kind of attack on each other as individuals.

During my elementary and secondary school experiences, the classmates routinely showed respect for one another. The love and appreciation continued up to and including today among my classmates that I grew up with in Austin, Texas. We were able to avoid distinctions on how one of us would be treated or respected based upon financial standing or whether a person was an athlete or in the band or other clubs or extracurricular affiliations. We were proud and respectful of all of those in our company as youth, and that has continued throughout adulthood. Each month our high school classmates gather to communicate on the telephone for a prayer session. We take the time to share prayers and thoughts of wisdom which each one of us may wish to share. The conversations are always respectful and caring, and we have never shared a negative comment about anyone.

I have incredibly positive thoughts and memories about my work environments. I have been fortunate to be surrounded by others whose professionalism and attitudes have been consistent with mine. Terms like excuse me, thank you, would you mind, I appreciate you and your contributions and please have been used commonly among colleagues throughout my interactions in the work environment. It has not been unusual for my colleagues to spend time at lunch or dinner inside and outside the office and issuing invitations for enjoying home meals together. Caution -- be careful in leadership not to require employees to eat during a multi-hour meeting, where food is brought in to save time, thereby, denying employees the break time away from the duties of the day. In my experience as employee, some of the most pleasant gatherings occurred during those break times where colleagues and I would leave the office building and enjoy lunch together outside of the office setting.

It is particularly important that each one of us shows respect for ourselves if we expect or want other people to show respect for us. Additionally, each one of us should make it a priority to show respect for other people. And always keep in mind the thought: <u>leave other people alone, except to be helpful</u>! Respect may be earned, but it is not ever legitimately given or received as the result of intimidation or based upon fear, demands or threats of harm. Practice!

Reader - Think; Share; Reflect: _____

_____

_____

15. Right way (over wrong) - It is not complicated. Do the right thing, regardless of the circumstances or what may appear to be a possible advantage to do otherwise. Doing the right thing enables you to enjoy the available benefits, while doing the wrong thing works in the opposite direction, short or long term. The decision to do right or wrong starts internally. If you must think about it, whether the action is right or wrong, always, always choose to do the "right" thing over wrong. The self-monitoring mechanisms inside should guide you in the right direction, with heavy reliance upon past experiences and an internal knowledge base in place to guide you. Practice!

➤ *Alignment with Bible Passages:*

"Therefore to him that knoweth to do good, and doeth *it* not, to him it is sin." (James 4: 17)

"For we know that the law is spiritual: but I am carnal, sold under sin. For that which I do I allow not: for what I would, that do I not; but what I hate, that do I. If then I do that which I would not, I consent unto the law that it *is* good. Now then it is no more I that do it, but sin that dwelleth in me . . . For the good that I would I do not: but the evil which I would not, that I do." (Romans 7: 14-17; 19)

"Be not overcome of evil, but overcome evil with good." (Romans 12: 21)

"Blessed *are* the peacemakers: for they shall be called the children of God. Blessed *are* they which are persecuted for righteousness' sake: for theirs is the kingdom of heaven. Blessed are ye, when *men* shall revile you, and persecute *you*, and shall say all manner of evil against you, falsely, for my sake. Rejoice, and be exceeding glad: for great is your reward in heaven: for so persecuted they the prophets which were before you." (Matthew 5: 9-12)

"Envyings, murders, drunkenness, revellings, and such like: of the which I tell you before, as I have also told *you* in time past, that they which do such things shall not inherit the kingdom of God. But the fruit of the Spirit is love, joy, peace, long-suffering, gentleness, goodness, faith, Meekness, temperance: against such there is no law." (Galatians 5: 21-23)

"Little children, let no man deceive you: he that doeth righteousness is righteous, even as he is righteous." (1 John 3: 7)

"For, brethren, ye have been called unto liberty; only *use* not liberty for an occasion to the flesh, but by love serve one another. For all the law is fulfilled in one word, *even* in this; Thou shalt love thy neighbour as thyself. But if ye bite and devour one another, take heed that ye be not consumed one of another." (Galatians 5: 13-15)

"And let us not be weary in well doing: for in due season we shall reap, if we faint not. As we have therefore opportunity, let us do good unto all *men*, especially unto them who are of the household of faith." (Galatians 6: 9-10)

"After this manner therefore pray ye: Our Father which art in heaven, Hallowed be thy name. Thy kingdom come. Thy will be done in earth, *as it is* in heaven. Give us this day our daily bread. And forgive us our debts, as we forgive our debtors. And lead us not into temptation, but deliver us from evil: For thine is the kingdom, and the power, and the glory, forever. Amen. For if ye forgive men their trespasses, your heavenly Father will also forgive you: But if ye forgive not men their trespasses, neither will your Father forgive your trespasses." (Matthew 6: 9-15)

"Be ye strong therefore, and let not your hands be weak: for your work shall be rewarded." (2 Chronicles 15: 7)

Reflection(s): "Let it go!" Let nothing and no one get in the way of your march toward greater success, and always remain goal directed and focused on "winning the game". Make sure all the "dots connect" in a rational manner and avoid blockages of progress by others or yourself. In stressful, tense, and emotional situations, time to practice WWWST concepts by using your head, not your mouth until you calm down. Practice: "Let it go!'

In life there will be times when you are faced with challenges for determining right from wrong in personal and professional environments. Even when others may encourage you to do the wrong thing, it is always better to choose right over wrong. This is especially important when the decisions are associated with moral, ethical, and legal issues. Examples of such issues are provided as follows: contract management; personnel actions; financial considerations; speed-limit driving and traffic laws; drugs and alcohol; bullying or bothering people; stealing.

Think about it in terms of consequences people face after an action is taken or in absence of a person doing the right thing -- consider risk-reward terms. You can count on it that someone else will know or find out about the situation and will tell someone else. It is a regular, normal occurrence that people want to talk, especially about those instances when they know of someone doing the wrong thing. It is always better when faced with decisions to do that which is right, period.

It is not just a matter of being practical. It is a matter of being careful, smart, and wise. You stand a much better chance of "winning the game" in sports and life when you follow the rules and do things the right way. You should, therefore, always consider what will happen when you operate out of bounds or contrary to what is right. You face being singled out by the game officials if involved in a sports activity and by law or work officials in cases of a law or policy violation. What follows then are consequences along with shame and humiliation, often, in public or social media reports.

I can vividly recall a situation where high school teachers in a central Texas school planned a science class field trip where the students would learn about nature during a river boat ride. Some students who happened to be cheerleaders and athletes participated in sneaking alcohol onto the boat and drinking during the boat ride. They were caught as one of the teachers observed empty beer cans being thrown into the water. The teachers reported the incident to school officials after the trip, and all students faced punishment following the trip. The punishment was strong, as a preventative measure and to demonstrate that even cheerleaders and athletes would face serious consequences for such violations. There were lots of discussions among parents of the students, central office and campus officials and community leaders, in disagreement about whether the punishments were fair or excessive. All of this could have been avoided if only the students had done the right thing in the first place. Regrettably, one of the contributing factors which led to the debate was that the students involved were active and popular students. Again, do the right thing and avoid such drama.

One strong measure of character is to observe a person's actions when he or she is faced with a decision to do the right thing, and the person is not aware of being watched. It is wise to believe that most often someone is watching your actions or will find out at some point. It should not matter, as doing the right thing is the better approach, even if difficult or unfavorable to you, personally. Practice!

Reader - Think; Share; Reflect: _____

_____

_____

16. Space (give, protect, stay in your lane) - It is most difficult to accurately determine whether someone wants or does not want a person in their "space" or near them. Better to "play it safe" and always be mindful that personal space is deserved by everyone. A violation of that privilege can often cause discomfort for them and you. Make sure you are "invited" in proximity, with no exceptions of leaving it to chance or guessing, if okay. If not sure of an invitation into another person's "space", keep a safe distance away from him or her. On the other hand, if you believe your private space is being violated, quietly move away to create a greater distance away from you, or simply inform the other person of your feeling of discomfort. Practice!

> *Alignment with Bible Passages:*

"The lines are fallen unto me in pleasant *places*; yea, I have a goodly heritage . . . I have set the LORD always before me: because *he is* at my right hand, I shall not be moved." (Psalm 16: 6; 8)

"With all lowliness and meekness, with long-suffering, forbearing one another in love; Endeavouring to keep the unity of the Spirit in the bond of peace." (Ephesians 4: 2-3)

"Let no corrupt communication proceed out of your mouth, but that which is good to the use of edifying, that it may minister grace unto the hearers." (Ephesians 4: 29)

"Finally, *be ye* all of one mind, having compassion one of another, love as brethren, *be* pitiful, *be* courteous: Not rendering evil for evil, or railing for railing: but contrariwise blessing; knowing that ye are thereunto called, that ye should inherit a blessing. For he that will love life, and see good days, let him refrain his tongue from evil, and his lips that they speak no guile: let him eschew evil, and do good; let him seek peace, and ensue it." (1 Peter 3: 8-11)

"To every *thing there is* a season, and a time to every purpose under the heaven: A time to be born, and a time to die; a time to plant, and a time to pluck up *that which* is planted; A time to kill, and a time to heal; a time to break down, and a time to build up; A time to weep, and a time to laugh; a time to mourn, and a time to dance; A time to cast away stones, and a time to gather stones together; a time to embrace, and a time to refrain from embracing; A time to get, and a time to lose; a time to keep, and a time to cast away; A time to rend, and a time to sew; a time to keep silence, and time to speak; A time to love, and a time to hate; a time of war, and a time of peace." (Ecclesiastes 3: 1-8)

"*Let your* conversation *be* without covetousness; *and be* content with such things as ye have: for he hath said, I will never leave thee, nor forsake thee. So that we may boldly say, The LORD is my helper, and I will not fear what man shall do unto me." (Hebrews 13: 5-6)

"Beware lest any man spoil you through philosophy and vain deceit, after the tradition of men, after the rudiments of the world, and not after Christ." (Colossians 2: 8)

"Ye have heard that it hath been said, Thou shalt love thy neighbour, and hate thine enemy. But I say unto you, Love your enemies, bless them that curse you, do good to them that hate you, and pray for them which despitefully use you, and persecute you." (Matthew 5: 43-44)

"And the King shall answer and say unto them, Verily I say unto you, Inasmuch as ye have done *it* unto one of the least of these my brethren, ye have done *it* unto me . . . Then shall he answer them, saying, Verily I say unto you, Inasmuch as ye did *it* not to one of the least of these, ye did *it* not to me." (Matthew 25: 40; 45)

"Owe no man any thing, but to love one another: for he that loveth another hath fulfilled the law. For this, Thou shalt not commit adultery, Thou shalt not kill, Thou shalt not steal, Thou shalt not bear false witness, Thou shalt not covet; *and if there be* any other commandment, it *is* briefly comprehended in this saying, namely, Thou shalt love thy neighbour as thyself. Love worketh no ill to his neighbour: therefore love *is* the fulfilling of the law." (Romans 13: 8-10)

Reflection(s): "Let it go!" Let nothing and no one get in the way of your march toward greater success, and always remain goal directed and focused on "winning the game". Make sure all the "dots connect" in a rational manner and avoid blockages of progress by others or yourself. In stressful, tense, and emotional situations, time to practice "stop talking" concepts by using your head, not your mouth until you calm down. Practice: "Let it go!"

The idea that there are times when a person just wants to be left alone is not a foreign or unique concept. It is a sense of reality which all of us wish to enjoy, some more often or less than others. There is a commonly accepted phrase, "Don't just do something, sit", or "Don't keep talking, be quiet – or stop talking". It is not just okay to be left alone, I believe it is a very natural experience. Whether the time is spent in reading, watching television or an activity or just taking time to relax or think, we all deserve and should take the time to enjoy our "space" without interruption. Therefore, it is also imperative that when it is not clear that your company is desired, let it go and move away.

Think of those times when a person may wish to dine alone. It is not unusual for another person to approach the person who is dining and make an offer to sit with him or her for the meal. They may approach the person and state, "I hate to see you sitting there eating alone". Guess what? There are times when a person wants and needs to enjoy the "space" and be left alone. The person who is alone should not be pressured to explain or be required to state a reason for the preference to be left to dine alone at that time.

I happen to be one of those who sometimes enjoys eating alone or with family, only. There are also times when I am comfortable with sharing mealtime with friends and associates. I can recall numerous times when someone approached me at work with an offer to take me out for dinner or lunch, at their cost. I have declined to accept those offers most of the time because such generosities result in an unwelcomed extension of the workday with the effect of taking away the time and opportunities for my preferred routine of eating alone or with family. Of course, I am always appreciative of genuine offers of hospitality. I believe it is important to protect my "space" relative to the time dedicated to personal preferences such as my own dining routines and those times dedicated for reading, meditation and thinking.

How about other times, such as while shopping, walking in the park, taking time to attend a program or watch a movie at the theatre or the idea of wanting to spend some "me" or "self" time at home? It should be left to the individual to determine whether to enjoy the time or space alone or with company. When a person indicates he or she wishes to be left alone is not time to automatically decide their state of mind or whether there is a problem. For example, there are many times when I just want to meditate or enjoy the time alone and not be interrupted or bothered by another person. In those instances, I would rather not talk on the telephone or engage in conversation with others. Of course, family time is more special and always welcomed.

Think about why there is conflict when a person is offended or feeling disrespected because another individual wants to be left alone. We should avoid making attempts to control another person through our words or actions. Just as importantly, we should not allow ourselves to become offended just because another person wishes to enjoy their space alone or in the company of others outside ourselves. Many conflicts may be avoided if we just follow a simple rule: "Better to 'play it safe' and be mindful that personal space is deserved by everyone." And, again, in thinking like a champion, we should all work at <u>leaving other people alone, except to be helpful</u>! Practice!

Reader - Think; Share; Reflect: _____

_____

_____

17. Teamwork (over self) - The concept of placing team or common good over self is one of the most cherished notions across the world. It is what is being practiced when, as a nation or church group or athletic team or any similar organization, the preferred standard is what is good for one is good for all. It has been said that "you cannot be almost on the team". You are on the team and act as such, or you are not really a full member of the group. Placing team over self is one of the most important principles of team sports and winning the game. It is also part of what drives the laws we live by and other rules which govern the common good. Practice!

➢ *Alignment with Bible Passages:*

"Two *are* better than one; because they have a good reward for their labour. For if they fall, the one will lift up his fellow: but woe to him *that is* alone when he falleth; for *he hath* not another to help him up. Again, if two lie together, then they have heat: but how can one be warm *alone*? And if one prevail against him, two shall withstand him; and a threefold cord is not quickly broken." (Ecclesiastes 4: 9-12)

"Now I beseech you, brethren, by the name of our Lord Jesus Christ, that ye all speak the same thing, and *that* there be no divisions among you; but *that* ye be perfectly joined together in the same mind and in the same judgment." (1 Corinthians 1: 10)

"And let us consider one another to provoke unto love and to good works: Not forsaking the assembling of ourselves together, as the manner of some *is*; but exhorting *one another*: and so much the more, as ye see the day approaching." (Hebrews 10: 24-25)

"BEHOLD, how good and how pleasant *it is* for brethren to dwell together in unity!" (Psalm 133:1)

"For as we have many members in one body, and all members have not the same office: So we *being* many, are one body in Christ, and every one members one of another." (Romans 12: 4-5)

"*Be* kindly affectioned one to another with brotherly love; in honour preferring one another." (Romans 12: 10)

"We then that are strong ought to bear the infirmities of the weak, and not to please ourselves. Let every one of us please *his* neighbour for *his* good to edification." (Romans 15: 1-2)

"Iron sharpeneth iron; so a man sharpeneth the countenance of his friend." (Proverbs 27: 17)

"*Let* nothing *be done* through strife or vainglory; but in lowliness of mind let each esteem other better than themselves. Look not every man on his own things, but every man also on the things of others." (Philippians 2: 3-4)

"As every man hath received the gift, *even so* minister the same to one another, as good stewards of the manifold grace of God." (1 Peter 4: 10)

Reflection(s): "Let it go!" Let nothing and no one get in the way of your march toward greater success, and always remain goal directed and focused on "winning the game". Make sure all the "dots connect" in a rational manner and avoid blockages of progress by others or yourself. In stressful, tense, and emotional situations, time to practice WWWST concepts by using your head, not your mouth until you calm down. Practice: "Let it go!"

Successful teams consistently demonstrate characteristics which are observable and well-practiced, where the concept of team is emphasized above self. Among other important strategies to achieve team success, it is critical to "connect the dots" in planning and in all phases of practicing and operating on a system approach, recognizing that all parts are interrelated. This concept is important for all teams: ballet, circus, sports teams, fine arts units, card players, family units, all other teams, and businesses. If, for example, practice is to start at 3:00 p.m., everyone on the team must arrive prior to 3:00 p.m. When the coach calls a play for the team to run during practice or a game, each person is responsible to do what is expected and to do it with great passion and effort. The president of an organization gives a directive to employees on how a report is to be written. When the report is completed and turned in, it should reflect what was directed. In an "own the store" mentality in business operations or school system, each person associated with the company should perform at the best of his or her talents and with a sense of strong "team" concept, realizing the product produced or outcomes can be only as good as the weakest link of workers' accomplishments.

While playing on the L. C. Anderson High School basketball team, we shouted a slogan prior to each game: "All for One – One for All!" We said those words loudly and with joy and commitment and meaning that we were proud members of the team and planned to operate as one. With those words we were acknowledging that what affected one of us affected all of us. We were also proclaiming that each one of us was committing our word to contributing as individuals in support of the team to win the game. Consider any team which is comprised of numerous "super" talented individuals, but they do not perform as champion teammates -- good, but not great. One quite common factor in such a situation is the lack of commitment to each other, and one or more members of the group tends to insist on placing his or her interests above that of the team.

The team concept naturally aligns with groups other than athletic teams. For example, consider work related organizations and departments, church groups, boy scouts and girl scouts' organizations, school clubs and more. The excellent teammates go beyond the words and practice and take actions that when the team is involved, it is not ever about "me", or "I", it is about what is best for the team. The work that goes into becoming an excellent marching band is strenuous, for example. It is not unusual for selection to be competitive and requiring a lot of hard work just to make the team. What follows is practice for hours and hours on playing the music and learning the routines and coordinating the steps and patterns for each performer to be on cue in playing the music and marching steps required. No excuses are acceptable, and during the live performances everyone who is present in the audience observes the level of excellence with joy, celebration, and approval or disappointment. The performance is accepted by the performers and audience only when and if the music is good and routines are well coordinated by all members of the band -- teamwork!

Winning is fun and losing is not. Excellent teams and businesses routinely enjoy an environment where each person in the organization is treated with respect and dignity, and they are made to feel valued. The people on the teams enjoy their work and being part of something special. Consider successful championship teams, such as the college football teams for the University of Alabama, and Clemson University. The coaches and players work hard at their craft, and they pay special, laser focus attention to details. They also make commitments to each other that they will execute their responsibility each play while on the playing field. And they have fun. For example, I recall observing the excitement among the Alabama football players during a practice meeting when superstar national basketball league player, Kobe Bryant (now deceased) visited and gave tips on thinking and acting like champions. I also observed several times following victories the Clemson University players and coaches enjoying dancing the "electric slide" in the dressing room -- well-coordinated and fun! The ideas of hard work and enjoyment are interjected into their programs and promoted in all communications among players, coaches, and other personnel.

Sometimes in leadership the simplest gestures can help with team building. For example, I can recall the enthusiasm when as principal at a middle school, I asked what would make the environment more pleasing, and the answer from the employees was they preferred brand-named toilet tissue. Asked and answered immediately by replacing the stock, system product with brand named products, specifically the brands preferred by the employees. In a similar move as superintendent in two separate school districts, I asked the employees their opinions on what would help to improve the work environment and strengthen morale, and the answer was they preferred the school calendar allow a full week off duty during the Thanksgiving Holidays -- Asked-answered! "Teamwork makes the dream work" is activated in live form and reality when those who are associated with team believe they are part of something special, they feel empowered and appreciated, and they are inspired beyond the words to do good for the team by what they see in the efforts of the leaders and each of their teammates. Practice!

Reader - Think; Share; Reflect: _____

_____

_____

18. Trustworthiness (trust, trusted) - The principle of trustworthiness is simple to understand but difficult for some to follow, either to trust or be trusted. When a person shares information or receives it, better that it remains among those who are directly engaged in the communication, written or verbal form. Whether the communication occurs among those in a small group of two or many more, it is important to practice the skills for trusting and being trustworthy.

➤ *Alignment with Bible Passages:*

"What shall we then say to these things? If God *be* for us, who *can be* against us? He that spared not his own Son, but delivered him up for us all, how shall he not with him also freely give us all things." (Romans 8: 31-32)

"In all things shewing thyself a pattern of good works: in doctrine *shewing* uncorruptness, gravity, sincerity, Sound speech, that cannot be condemned; that he that is of the contrary part may be ashamed, having no evil thing to say of you . . . For the grace of God that bringeth salvation hath appeared to all men, Teaching us that, denying ungodliness and worldly lusts, we should live soberly, righteously, and godly, in this present world." (Titus 2: 7-8; 11-12)

"He that walketh uprightly walketh surely: but he that perverteth his ways shall be known." (Proverbs 10: 9)

"A talebearer revealeth secrets: but he that is of a faithful spirit concealeth the matter." (Proverbs 11:13)

"Better *is* the poor that walketh in his uprightness, than *he that is* perverse *in his* ways, though he *be* rich." (Proverbs 28: 6)

"Be not deceived: evil communications corrupt good manners." (1 Corinthians 15: 33)

"Thy word *is* true *from* the beginning: and every one of thy righteous judgments *endureth* forever." (Psalm 119: 160)

"These *are* the things that ye shall do; Speak ye every man the truth to his neighbour; execute the judgment of truth and peace in your gates: And let none of you imagine evil in your hearts against his neighbour; and love no false oath: for all these *are things* I hate, saith the LORD." (Zechariah 8: 16-17)

"Lie not one to another, seeing that ye have put off the old man with his deeds; And have put on the new *man*, which is renewed in knowledge after the image of him that created him." (Colossians 3: 9-10)

"Sanctify them through thy truth: thy word is truth." (John 17: 17)

Reflection(s): "Let it go!" Let nothing and no one get in the way of your march toward greater success, and always remain goal directed and focused on "winning the game". Make sure all the "dots connect" in a rational manner and avoid blockages of progress by others or yourself. In stressful, tense, and emotional situations, time to practice WWWST concepts by using your head, not your mouth until you calm down. Practice: "Let it go!"

Question: Whether to trust or decide not to trust others and whether to operate as trustworthy or not, and to what extent? These are questions we all routinely face in communication with others. It is not unusual for a person to want to trust others, especially among those who are often around in proximity -- friends and loved ones. There are times when the decision on whether a person can be trusted is based upon current circumstances or situations and other times when the determination is based upon multiple years of awareness. Once it is determined that a person is not to be trusted, that decision is exceedingly difficult to overcome, especially if the matter involves dishonesty.

It has been said that you should not trust anyone fully without question, or to trust only close family members and, even then, trust on a limited basis. At the least be careful to limit trust to those of whom you are convinced have earned it. Likewise, it is important that each of us is conscious about being trustworthy, within and across business and personal relationships. It is a choice. There are some simple and doable traits that each of us can actively demonstrate: be honest and honorable all times; love one another as self and be willing to show it, noting that in love relationships each person is trustworthy and loyal; be integrous always; and think and do the right thing within and across all groups in communications.

Unfortunately, there are people who will routinely "smile in your face" and, later, demonstrate that those smiles were phony, at best, and at times they will take actions that turn out to be vengeful and hateful. They are quick to sabotage when out of site. It is better not to spend time trying to convince these types of people about right and wrong or to exert energy attempting to make them like or respect you. It is they who may or may not realize some day the value of trustworthiness, professionalism, honor, and friendship and not you; again, it is a choice one makes to be trustworthy or not.

Can a person be almost trustworthy, or trustworthy on some days and not on other days? No -- almost trustworthiness is not realistic. How about a person being trustworthy around some people and not around others? Again, the idea of a person being almost trustworthy is an example of a person who is not to be trusted by anyone. Putting it another way, it is inadvisable to trust a person who is honest, honorable, and reliable only on an "on call" or situational basis. Better to start with trusting only those who have earned such an honor. And it is highly predicable that some will not be so favored. A person who is trustworthy will always show concern for your well-being and that of their own, and you can count on them, when things are not going well and even when no one is looking. Practice!

Reader - Think; Share; Reflect: _____

_____

_____

19. Weapons Free (compliant legally) - Think and do everything in your power to avoid a lifestyle of being around or using illegal weapons. There are rules for recreational hunting and self-defense which, when applied to specified situations, are acceptable in society. These rules do not fit in any way if the intent in possession or use of weapons may cause unprovoked harm to self or others. Think, plan, act responsibly by following the law and the standards for "doing unto others" what you would expect and desire, if you were confronted with the same situation. Practice!

➤ *Alignment with Bible Passages*:

"No weapon that is formed against thee shall prosper; and every tongue *that* shall rise against thee in judgment thou shalt condemn. This is the heritage of the servants of the LORD, and their righteousness *is* of me, saith the LORD." (Isaiah 54: 17)

"Ye have heard that it hath been said, An eye for an eye, and a tooth for a tooth. But I say unto you, That ye resist not evil: but whosoever shall smite thee on thy right cheek, turn to him the other also." (Matthew 5: 38-39)

"Then said Jesus unto him, Put up again thy sword into his place: for all they that take the sword shall perish with the sword." (Matthew 26: 52)

"Finally, my brethren, be strong in the Lord, and in the power of his might. Put on the whole armor of God, that ye may be able to stand against the wiles of the devil. For we wrestle not against flesh and blood, but against principalities, against powers, against the rulers of the darkness of this world, against spiritual wickedness in high *places*." (Ephesians 6: 10-12)

"If it be possible, as much as lieth in you, live peaceably with all men . . .

Be not overcome of evil, but overcome evil with good." (Romans 12: 18; 21)

"Be strong and courageous, be not afraid nor dismayed for the king of Assyria, nor for all the multitude that *is* with him: for *there be* more with us than with him: With him *is* an arm of flesh; but with us *is* the LORD our God to help us, and to fight our battles. And the people rested themselves upon the words of Hezekiah king of Judah." (2 Chronicles 32: 7-8)

"There is no king saved by the multitude of an host: a mighty man is not delivered by much strength. An horse *is* a vain thing for safety: neither shall he deliver *any* by his great strength. Behold, the eye of the LORD *is* upon them that fear him, upon them that hope in his mercy." (Psalm 33: 16-18)

"He delighteth not in the strength of the horse: he taketh not pleasure in the legs of a man. The LORD taketh pleasure in them that fear him, in those that hope in his mercy." (Psalm 147: 10-11)

"Then was Jesus led up of the Spirit into the wilderness to be tempted of the devil . . . And when the tempter came to him, he said, if thou be the Son of God, command that these stones be made bread. But he answered and said, It is written, Man shall not live by bread alone, but by every word that proceedeth out of the mouth of God." (Matthew 4: 1, 3-4)

"Then said David to the Philistine, Thou comest to me with a sword, and with a spear, and with a shield: but I come to thee in the name of the LORD of hosts, the God of the armies of Israel, whom thou hast defied." (1 Samuel 17: 45)

Reflection(s): "Let it go!" Let nothing and no one get in the way of your march toward greater success, and always remain goal directed and focused on "winning the game". Make sure all the "dots connect" in a rational manner and avoid blockages of progress by others or yourself. In stressful, tense, and emotional situations, time to practice WWWST concepts by using your head, not your mouth until you calm down. Practice: "Let it go!"

Always keep in mind the thought: "Leave other people alone, except to be helpful!" Think about how many incidents and conflicts and violence could have been avoided if those involved had practiced this point: "Leave other people alone, except to be helpful!" Mind your own business and stay out of the business of others is another way of putting it. Still another common and impactful phrase is the following: Treat others as you wish to be treated. Some conflicts are unavoidable or, at the least, difficult to prevent. The better path toward resolution is to talk it out, including listening to the points of view of others and giving serious consideration to those ideas. Then use common sense in response and no weapons to resolve conflicts.

The possession of weapons may give a person a sense of comfort for prevention against harm. Also, weapons may be used in a reasonable manner for hunting. Weapons, however, should not be used in violence perpetrated upon another person or oneself. The use of a weapon is often a final act that cannot be reversed. In anger it is always better to walk away and cool off and not to attempt to resolve or address the problem at that exact time. It is really that simple; just walk away and deal with the situation later once you have had a chance to cool off. Too often it becomes a matter of pride and finding it important to demonstrate that you are not afraid, and you want to prove you will not be intimidated. No! Walk away rather than allow yourself to get caught in a situation where violence or serious argument will be the result of your communication. Likewise, there is no good time or reason to intimidate another person or to bully a person into submission as a means for resolving conflict. If you are a person who may tend to have a problem with quick anger and problems with patience, you should not carry weapons on your person or in a vehicle in which you are riding -- too easy to allow anger to overpower your sense of purpose and ability to avoid the temptation to use the weapon to settle your differences.

Do you know someone or people who were directly affected by weapons violence, either as the victim or perpetrator? For most if not all the answer to that question is, regrettably, yes. And so often in these situations the resulting impact from the act of weapons violence is long-lasting and memorable but the act itself or associated drama lasts only a few seconds or minutes. If only one of those involved would have walked away and allowed themselves to cool off or had made the decision not become involved in the first place, the violent act would have been prevented. I can recall visiting a school in California as part of an education program tour. The tour guide pointed out a board which was hanging on the wall at the entrance that had names of youth lost to violence; so sad the long list of names posted. It was a vivid reminder of what happens when bad choices are made, and the violence is not avoided. The good news during the tour was that most of the students in the school were alive were doing well. Yet, good is not great, and one loss to acts of violence is too many, let alone the many such losses each year within and across the nation and, indeed, the world. Avoid the use of weapons through keeping your cool and walking away when things begin to get "heated" in communication. A weapons free lifestyle can make the difference in saving a life, including your own. Walk away. Practice: "Let it go!"

Reader - Think; Share; Reflect: _____

_____

_____

20. (WWWST) What to say, when to say it and when to stop talking - In communication begin with and maintain a smile on your face throughout the conversation or presentation. Be factual, avoid speculation and always be honest and accurate in each comment made. It is best to avoid saying "no comment", as it may imply you are hiding something. No excuses or whining and do not seek pity, and never speak when angry. Calm down first and do not say what you are thinking if unhappy. It is

important not to make comments about someone who is not present. If not well prepared for the subject, delay until another time or delegate the task of responding to someone else who may be better able to respond. If you do not know a good response, say that you do not know. When in doubt or when you have already sufficiently addressed the mission or topic, stop talking. Better not to say it if not sure whether you should. Again, keep smiling. Practice!

➤ *Alignment with Bible Passages*:

"And that ye study to be quiet, and to do your own business, and to work with your own hands, as we commanded you. That ye may walk honestly toward them that are without, and *that* ye may have lack of nothing." (1 Thessalonians 4: 11-12)

"And the same day, when the even was come, he saith unto them, Let us pass over unto the other side. And when they had sent away the multitude, they took him even as he was in the ship. And there were also with him other little ships. And there arose a great storm of wind, and the waves beat into the ship, so that it was now full. And he was in the hinder part of the ship, asleep on a pillow: and they awake him, and say unto him, Master, carest thou not that we perish? And he arose, and rebuked the wind, and said unto the sea, Peace, be still. And the wind ceased, and there was a great calm. And he said unto them, Why are ye so fearful? how is it that ye have no faith? (Mark 4: 35-40)

"Finally, brethren, farewell. Be perfect, be of good comfort, be of one mind, live in peace; and the God of love and peace shall be with you." (2 Corinthians: 13: 11)

"And say unto him, Take heed, and be quiet; fear not, neither be faint-hearted for the two tails of these smoking firebrands, for the fierce anger of Rezin with Syria, and of the son of Remaliah." (Isaiah 7: 4)

"A Soft answer turneth away wrath: but grievous words stir up anger." (Proverbs 15: 1)

"A wholesome tongue *is* a tree of life: but perverseness therein *is* a breach in the spirit . . . The lips of the wise disperse knowledge: but the heart of the foolish *doeth* not so." (Proverbs 15: 4; 7)

"Set a watch, O LORD, before my mouth; keep the door of my lips." (Psalm 141: 3)

"A time to rend, and a time to sew; a time to keep silence, and a time to speak." (Ecclesiastes 3: 7)

"Not that which goeth into the mouth defileth a man; but that which cometh out of the mouth, this defileth a man." (Matthew 15: 11)

"Wherefore, my beloved brethren, let every man be swift to hear, slow to speak, slow to wrath." (James 1: 19)

Reflection(s): "Let it go!" Let nothing and no one get in the way of your march toward greater success, and always remain goal directed and focused on "winning the game". Make sure all the "dots connect" in a rational manner and avoid blockages of progress by others or yourself. In stressful, tense, and emotional situations, time to practice WWWST concepts by using your head, not your mouth until you calm down. Practice: "Let it go!"

The bottom line is thinking before you speak and determining prior to speaking whether the comment adds value to the conversation or not. It matters in every conversation what you say, when to say it and when it is better to hold on to the comment and leave it unspoken. Far too often people tend to operate otherwise and speak without thinking and say too much -- too late! Stop it; better for us to practice listening more and talking less.

A few examples follow -- still long way to go for needed changes and growth in the attitudes of people. One noticeably clear example of how important it is to think before you comment is the situation in the year 2018 which resulted in the resignation of a Texas school superintendent, following his "posting" on Facebook a response to an online newspaper story where he was critical of the quarterback of the Houston Texans football team, stating among other things, "You can't count on a black quarterback." He resigned, expressing in his resignation letter his deepest apologies for making such a comment -- too late! He also stated that the comments were wrong and inappropriate. So true. He apologized directly to the quarterback for his remarks in a public statement, and he expressed appreciation to the quarterback for not criticizing or belittling him for his remarks, choosing instead peace and positivity. Of course, beyond the mistake of making the original, offensive public statement of this nature, also troubling was the attitude and ignorance displayed, especially by an educator in a position of leadership. This incident could easily have been avoided by thinking before acting about what to say, when to say it and when to stop talking.

Another situation involved a radio host in 2007 in a program simulcast on a television station, where the host made the comment to look at those "nappy-headed hos" (whores) in referring to an exceptionally talented, successful women's basketball team. The comment was made after another radio personality called the team "hardcore hos" (whores). The show was cancelled shortly following the program. A Georgia superintendent faced discipline and later resigned in 2018 following release of an audio recording filled with racist rants, including use of the term "nigger" and other derogatory comments about construction workers. Another case where attitude matters and demonstration of why it is better to think before speaking and to know what to say, when to say it and when to stop talking.

Still another example of a person speaking before thinking involved the general manager of a major league baseball team in 1987, where during a public television interview in responding to a question about why there are not more black baseball managers, he stated that "I truly believe that they may not have some of the necessities to be, let's say, a field manager, or perhaps a general manager." The interview host asked whether he really believed that, and the general manager stated, "Well, I don't say that all of them, but they certainly are short. How many quarterbacks do you have? How many pitchers do you have that are black?" And he went on to say that black athletes are not good swimmers because they do not have the buoyancy... and more. Stop it; stop talking if not appropriate and helpful to self or others. In the year 2020 many of the residents and students in a school district in the state of Texas were embarrassed following a ruling by the school principal (and supported by the central administration) that a senior high school student of color was required to get a haircut because of the length of his hair and the dreadlocks style. The student was suspended and told that if he did not cut his hair, he would not be allowed to participate in the senior prom or graduation ceremony. The story was reported on national news amid complaints from the family that the decision was discriminatory, as the hair style was part of his family heritage and noting that the student had attended the school for several years without problems and had made good grades. The story was broadcast nationally. Due to national attention and strong disagreement with the ruling, the student received a large scholarship from a celebrity and attended the 92nd Academy Awards show in California as guests of the producers of an Oscar nominated short film about hair. The school district's reactions to the situation came across as arrogant, insensitive and tone deaf as well as backwards, especially given the diverse composition of the student body and criticisms by students not of color that they had not faced the same consequences. The student decided to transfer to a different school district. Those involved in handling the situation could have benefited by paying more attention to what to say, when to say it and when to stop talking.

It is quite common, and we can all recall instances where we wished the person talking would stop. Whether such occurrences involved a formal presentation or casual conversation, church sermon, school speech, television or radio interview or report, or business meeting, in these moments it may seem that the end of the talk was long awaited by all. We routinely forget or ignore the common rules of speaking, for example:

- Think before speaking.
- Make the point succinctly, then pause.
- Connect the sentences in a paragraph and include a topic, middle substance and ending.
- Know the facts and, in general, what you are speaking about before you open your mouth.
- Never speak when angry and show no frowning in public.
- Know your audience and communicate with them, not to them.
- Do not complain about someone who is not in the conversation.
- Listen. Stop talking.

I have developed a routine that if I stop listening before you stop talking, I will disengage and move away from the presentation or conversation. Otherwise, it turns into a distraction, and no one wishes to experience distraction by choice. I choose not to be bored or distracted, for sure. I also will routinely ask during presentations that if the audience stops listening before I stop speaking to please let me know so that I can adjust or end the presentation. Fortunately, to date I have not been faced with such a scenario. Think of those instances when you thought after making a remark you wished you could take it back, unsaid? It is always, always better to think first and then speak. Pausing to think during the conversation is not only not a problem but a skill which when mastered can be helpful.

Among the many challenges during doctoral studies at The University of Texas at Austin, one of the intriguing exercises was to make presentations within a brief, designated period, ten minutes or so to make your case. It was a highly effective practice for polishing our skills for making effective presentations. Practice!

Reader - Think; Share; Reflect – think of other examples of helpful tips on what to say, when to say it, and when to stop talking.

21. Zero bullying (allowed, initiated, or involvement and no fighting) - Treat everyone as you wish to be treated every day, period! Better to forgive and forget than to retaliate or get even. No time to hold grudges and no victory in overpowering or deliberately being mean to another person. Practice the skills for learning from the past, enjoying the present and looking forward to the future. Learn the skills for forgiving. "Hanging on" to the past is a waste of time and helps no one, including you. Anger is an emotion which can be controlled, remembering if they anger you by the things they say or do, they have "conquered" you. Practice!

➤ *Alignment with Bible Passages*:

"Thou shalt not avenge, nor bear any grudge against the children of thy people, but thou shalt love thy neighbour as thyself: I *am* the LORD." (Leviticus 19: 18)

"FRET not thyself because of evildoers, neither be thou envious against workers of iniquity. For they shall soon be cut down like the grass, and wither as the green herb. Trust in the LORD, and do good; *so* shalt thou dwell in the land, and verily thou shalt be fed. Delight thyself also in the LORD; and he shall give thee the desires of thine heart . . . Cease from anger, and forsake wrath: fret not thyself in any wise to do evil. For evildoers shall be cut off: but those that wait upon the LORD, they shall inherit the earth." (Psalm 37: 1-4; 8-9)

"Recompense to no man evil for evil. Provide things honest in the sight of all men. If it be possible, as much as lieth in you, live peaceably with all men." (Romans 12: 17-18)

"These six *things* doth the LORD hate; yea, seven *are* an abomination unto him. A proud look, a lying tongue, and hands that shed innocent blood, An heart that deviseth wicked imaginations, feet that be swift in running to mischief,

A false witness *that* speaketh lies, and he that soweth discord among brethren." (Proverbs 6: 16 – 19)

"A soft answer turneth away wrath: but grievous words stir up anger." (Proverbs 15: 1)

"Whoso rewardeth evil for good, evil shall not depart from his house. The beginning of strife *is as* when one letteth out water: therefore leave off contention, before it be meddled with." (Proverbs 17: 13-14)

"Ye have heard that it hath been said, Thou shalt love thy neighbour, and hate thine enemy. But I say unto you, Love your enemies, bless them that curse you, do good to them that hate you, and pray for them which despitefully use you, and persecute you; That ye may be the children of your Father which is in heaven: for he maketh his sun to rise on the evil and on the good, and sendeth rain on the just and on the unjust. For if ye love them which love you, what reward have ye? Do not even the publicans the same? And if ye salute your brethren only, what do ye more than others? Do not even the publicans so? Be ye therefore perfect, even as your Father which is in heaven is perfect." (Matthew 5: 43-48)

"The golden rule. Therefore all things whatsoever ye would that men should do to you, do ye even so to them: for this is the law and the prophets." (Matthew 7: 12)

"Let no corrupt communication proceed out of your mouth, but that which is good to the use of edifying, that it may minister grace unto the hearers." (Ephesians 4: 29)

"And thou shalt love the LORD thy God with all thy heart, and with all thy soul, and with all thy mind, and with all thy strength: this *is* the first commandment. And the second *is* like, *namely* this, Thou shalt love thy neighbour as thyself.

There is none other commandment greater than these."
(Mark 12: 30-31)

Reflection(s): "Let it go!" Let nothing and no one get in the way of your march toward greater success, and always remain goal directed and focused on "winning the game". Make sure all the "dots connect" in a rational manner and avoid blockages of progress by others or yourself. In stressful, tense, and emotional situations, time to practice WWWST concepts by using your head, not your mouth until you calm down. Practice: "Let it go!"

There is no good reason to bully or intimidate another person. Everyone deserves to live in peace and freedom from harm, verbal and physical. It is not only important not to bully or harm, but also important that each one of us reaches out to help others, as a high priority. With wide use of social media, bullying is more of a common occurrence than before. Such cowardly behavior can be perpetrated from afar but is still just as hurtful and harmful.

I am proud of and thankful for the lessons learned in growing up, especially at home. My parents were consistent and repetitive in reminding my brothers and sisters and me during childhood and beyond that we should always help and not harm other people. Those lessons were consistently promoted in the neighborhood among our adult neighbors, teachers, and ministers.

There are circumstances where those you may wish to assist would rather go it alone. That is, the act of reaching out to help others is only appreciated as helpful when it is welcomed by the recipient of such offers. And, again, the act of bullying another person may come across as verbal – or non-verbal (appearance of ignoring a person), and it may be physical. A person should not push themselves upon others, even in offers to be helpful.

I can recall numerous instances while growing up as a child and in adulthood, observing comments and acts of kindness. I have also observed the opposite, including conduct, which was unwelcomed, crude, and disrespectful of others and bullying. Fortunately, the acts of kindness in my experience and observations far exceed that of any other conduct. In fact, I am proud of and thankful for having the attitude of gaining joy and happiness when I observe others enjoying happiness and joy -- it can be infectious, indeed.

And always keep in mind the thought: <u>Leave other people alone, except to be helpful</u>! Practice!

Reader - Think; Share; Reflect: _____

_____

_____

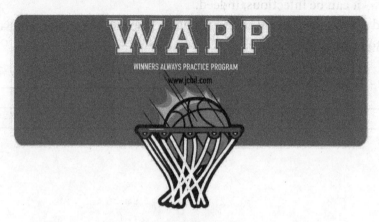

What To Say And When To Stop Talking

Common Sense
Continuous Improvement
Discipline
Focus
Follow Law
Healthy Lifestyle
Honesty
Honor
Listening
Love
Loyalty
Protect Property
Reading
Respect
Right Way
Space
Teamwork
Trustworthiness
Weapons Free
Zero Bullying

Logo - Author and Mary (Brown) Ruegg;
Chart - Darchase Designs

————————————— *Part Two* —————————————

WAPP List of Components and Definitions

Twenty-one easy-to-address behaviors, practices, qualities and areas of growth and development to win -- in games and life. By practicing all day everyday each of these categories, the chances to win increases in all phases of life, games, school and for getting along with others within and across race, class and otherwise. Yes, we can all succeed and get along with others if we want to and practice toward perfection in the following, well established and accepted behaviors, and practices, as provided not including biblical alignments and and reflections:

1. Common sense -- Common sense relates to natural tendencies and knowledge based upon routine growth experiences. The information "bank" to "pull from" or benefit from is common to all, and special training and experiences are not required for reference in determining how best to behave. Or, stated in more common terms, act like you are smart or well trained and dignified, especially, if others are around or may be affected by your behavior. Always avoid behaving "stupidly" when it is just as easy to behave "smartly." Practice!

2. Continuous improvement - No one is perfect, and everyone can and should strive to improve. Part of the human growth and development experience is that natural changes occur over which we have no control. Regarding those things over which we do have control, it is imperative to plan for and take advantage of opportunities to improve, within and across all forms of knowledge and conduct. It is safe to say that a person is on the incline in growth and development or in decline, as nothing in the human existence remains the same, over time. Never, ever give up or quit. Practice!

3. Discipline - Self-discipline is about making choices that are controlled by only one person, that is you! It is one of the most important decisions and, yet, too often one of the most challenging to manage. When managed effectively you stay out of trouble and avoid being confronted with problems and circumstances which can easily become a distraction and block progress toward happiness and well-being. Practice!

4. Focus - It is so easy to set goals and, yet, much more difficult to focus and set plans for and take the actions that are necessary to achieve them. Focusing entails controlling thoughts and actions to address with laser like attention on what matters the most. To focus is also not allowing distractions that may delay or prevent the outcomes desired. You can always find some reason not to focus and many better reasons to focus and maintain it, regardless of the temptations to do otherwise. Practice!

5. Follow Law - Laws exist for a reason: to protect all from harm, promote democracy and support us all as we seek to enjoy the "common good" and better quality of life. Do what you are supposed to do and not what you are not. Always keep the brain "open", and keep the thoughts and actions directed toward advantages for and reasons to follow all laws whether local, state or nationally generated. There is always a possibility of being caught, thereby, bringing negative attention toward you and

penalties which can derail or ruin the "road" to winning on and off the playing field or court. Remember, in the "world" of current technology, officials can find out all kinds of information through review of records from cameras, cell phones, credit cards and banking records. Sooner or later when you fail to follow the law, you will be caught and will face the consequences of your actions. Practice!

6. Healthy lifestyle (no alcohol, drugs, eat right & exercise) - Being healthy is directly affected and driven by lifestyle and choices about eating, drinking, exercising, resting, and intake of substances. Attitude makes a difference realizing, for example, that expending the energy for a smile is far less difficult to develop than to develop a frown, and the impact is more healthful. To smile and seek happiness and acting out such an emotion is a good idea. Remember, how you live your life is your decision and none is more important than to choose to live a healthy lifestyle. Practice!

7. Honor (think and act your best with integrity and character) – Everyone has a name. That "good name" represents your family, self, and history -- past and future. The best way to protect that "good name" is to think and act with integrity and strong character. Such behavior is expected and preferred in all circles of life across the world, characterized by carrying oneself and treating others with respect and dignity and in accordance with the law and "high" moral character. Practice!

8. Honesty - Tell the truth and think, act, and live truthfully in all communications and transactions. Honesty is important whether related to the commission or omission of actions or comments in pursuance of the truth. Even in cases where the truth is not apparent or may be hidden from open view or misunderstood, the best approach is to "fill in the blanks" for accuracy rather than to allow misperceptions or lack of access to truth to prevail. Practice!

9. Listening - To listen is a major component in communication and is as important as speaking. There is a major difference in hearing and listening. Hearing simply perceives the sounds, while listening requires hearing the sounds and applying what is heard to a sense of meaning and determining an appropriate response, if any. Hearing is a natural function of the body in acknowledgement of sound; listening requires thinking and action. Practice!

10. Love (give and seek over hatred) - To love and be loved are equally important and a significant part of enjoying a successful lifestyle. Love, in a real sense, is connected within and across every emotion, thought and action; although, you cannot see it and touch it. It is always there. Each one of us wants to be loved and appreciated, and each one of us has the innate ability to give and receive love. There is no room or good time in a "high quality" lifestyle for hatred, either to spread, devote time to it in thoughts or actions, or to experience it. Practice!

11. Loyalty - Loyalty is an important factor for achieving a common goal. Once the members of the group are identified and the group norms are established, there is an expectation of loyalty or agreement with all members of the team or group. Membership will change over time, with new members added and others leaving the group. Once norms are clear and established and there is a goal in mind for winning or high achievement, everyone has to believe in and practice the concept of counting on other members of the group and being counted upon, as a loyal or committed member of the group. Practice!

12. Protect property (of self and others and not steal) - It is not complicated. There is no good reason to steal or even think about it. Besides being the wrong thing to do by law and violation in morality, stealing is hurtful to both self and others. It does not matter that no one is around to see you steal; it is just as wrong. At the same time, it is important to plan for and take actions to

protect one's own property. Take steps even as simple as keeping keys or wallet in the same, exact place while traveling or sleeping or locking the door behind you for safety and protection of property. Think, plan, practice!

13. Reading - Reading is basic to all other knowledge, and it is key to all learning and the "spine" which holds everything together. If you cannot read, everybody will know it. Also, there is no "victory" in being illiterate. When you speak, your speech is a clear and public indicator of your level of preparation and intelligence. Reading is a means to acquire more tools and information for excellent communication skills. A person who is a poor or reluctant reader shows his or her lack of preparation and obvious unwillingness to grow in the skill set required for a good fit in society. You have a choice whether to be viewed as intelligent or unintelligent and, like any other skill set, you must practice each day to improve. Practice!

14. Respect (self and others and mind your business) - You deserve to be respected and so does everyone else. Respect starts with self and how you think and act and is apparent in all you say and do. It is far better to demonstrate positive regard toward others than to leave interpretation of your intent to chance. It is also important to give and receive respectful gestures and non-verbal cues in communication with other people. When confronted with decisions on whether to get involved or not, better to mind your own business, especially if the issue is not of your direct concern. Stay out of it. Practice!

15. Right way (over wrong) - It is not complicated. Do the right thing, regardless of the circumstances or what may appear to be a possible advantage to do otherwise. Doing the right thing enables you to enjoy the available benefits, while doing the wrong thing works in the opposite direction, short or long term. The decision to do right or wrong starts internally. If you must think about it, whether the action is right or wrong, always, always

choose to do the "right" thing over wrong. The self-monitoring mechanisms inside should guide you in the right direction, with heavy reliance upon past experiences and an internal knowledge base in place to guide you. Practice!

16. Space (give, protect, stay in your lane) - It is most difficult to accurately determine whether someone wants or does not want a person in their "space" or near them. Better to "play it safe" and always be mindful that personal space is deserved by everyone. A violation of that privilege can often cause discomfort for them and you. Make sure you are "invited" in proximity, with no exceptions of leaving it to chance or guessing, if okay. If not clear of an invitation into another person's "space", keep a safe distance away from him or her. And if you believe your private space is being violated, quietly move away to create a greater distance away from you, or simply inform the other person of your feeling of discomfort. Practice!

17. Teamwork (over self)—The concept of placing team or common good over self is one of the most cherished notions across the world. It is what is being practiced when, as a nation or church group or athletic team or any similar organization, the preferred standard is what is good for one is good for all. It has been said that "you cannot be almost on the team". You are on the team and act as such, or you are not really a full member of the group. Placing team over self is one of the most important principles of team sports and winning the game. It is also part of what drives the laws we live by and other rules which govern the common good. Practice!

18. Trustworthiness (trust, trusted) - The principle of trustworthiness is simple to understand but difficult for some to follow, either to trust or be trusted. When a person shares information or receives it, better that it remains among those who are directly engaged in the communication, written or verbal form. Whether the communication occurs among those

in a small group of two or many more, it is important to practice the skills for trusting and being trustworthy.

19. Weapons Free (compliant legally) - Think and do everything in your power to avoid a lifestyle of being around or using illegal weapons. There are rules for recreational hunting and self-defense which, when applied to specified situations, are acceptable in society. These rules do not fit in any way if the intent in possession or use of weapons may cause unprovoked harm to self or others. Think, plan, act responsibly by following the law and the standards for "doing unto others" what you would expect and desire, if you were confronted with the same situation. Practice!

20. (WWWST) What to say, when to say it and when to stop talking - In communication begin with and maintain a smile on your face throughout the conversation or presentation. Be factual, avoid speculation and always be honest and accurate in each comment made. It is best to avoid saying "no comment", as it may imply you are hiding something. No excuses or whining and do not seek pity, and never speak when angry. Calm down first and do not say what you are thinking if unhappy. It is important not to make comments about someone who is not present. If not well prepared for the subject, delay until another time or delegate the task of responding to someone else who may be better able to respond. If you do not know a good response, say that you do not know. When in doubt or when you have already sufficiently addressed the mission or topic, stop talking. Better not to say it if not sure whether you should. And, again, keep smiling. Practice!

21. Zero bullying (allowed, initiated, or involvement and no fighting) - Treat everyone as you wish to be treated every day, period! Better to forgive and forget than to retaliate or get even. No time to hold grudges and no victory in overpowering or deliberately being mean to another person. Practice the skills for

learning from the past, enjoying the present and looking forward
to the future. Learn the skills for forgiving. "Hanging on" to the
past is a waste of time and helps no one, including you. Anger
is an emotion which can be controlled, remembering if they
anger you by the things they say or do, they have "conquered"
you. Practice!

--- *Part Three* ---

Conclusion

This book addresses some human behaviors and activities which everyone can achieve successfully. That is, every component of the Winners Always Practice Program can be successfully achieved each day by every person. And age is not a determining factor on the level of achievement attainable -- from young child to mature adult to senior citizen. It does not matter which country, state, city, or neighborhood a person is in, the best route for high quality of life for all is for all to behave in a positive manner.

In life every human is as important as another. No matter the race or financial standing, we are all equal and imperfect in our thoughts and actions and prone to make mistakes. No one is better or more important than another person. Some of the more important skills and actions we take in our routine activities are simple to accomplish. It is desirable and more comfortable to always practice these guiding thoughts for a harmonious and positive lifestyle. For example, you:

- Are nice, thoughtful, and friendly in interactions with other people.
- Take time routinely to help someone or group of people.
- Think about and take actions for serving the "common good" over self-interests.

- Apply the principles for using common sense, always taking time to think before acting and for avoiding foolish things.
- Take steps to continue to improve in all behaviors, realizing that great is better than good, and excellent is better than acceptable or average.
- Focus with laser-like attention on that which is important.
- Demonstrate self-discipline within and across all activities in your daily routines.
- Know how to "let it go" when faced with situations over which you do not have control and which occurred in the past, especially when nothing is gained.
- Dream for a better way for achieving self and common interests and for setting goals and designing plans required for success in accomplishing them.
- Are always honest, honorable, loyal, respectful, trustworthy in style and substance not some of the time, but all the time.
- Always follow the law and make it a practice not to bother other people, except to be helpful.
- Live a healthy and happy lifestyle, full of love and appreciation for self and others.
- Listen keenly to others while speaking.
- Acknowledge and appreciate the team concept and contribute toward assuring roles and responsibilities are addressed by all concerned.
- Vote in elections.
- Have confidence, believe in self, and keep the faith.

If....

By Rudyard Kipling
(1895)

If you can keep your head when all about you
Are losing theirs and blaming it on you;
If you can trust yourself when all men doubt you,
But make allowance for their doubting too;
If you can wait and not be tired by waiting,
Or, being lied about, don't deal in lies,
Or being hated don't give way to hating,
And yet don't look too good, nor talk too wise:

If you can dream — and not make dreams your master;
If you can think — and not make thoughts your aim;
If you can meet with Triumph and Disaster
And treat those two impostors just the same;
If you can bear to hear the truth you've spoken
Twisted by knaves to make a trap for fools,
Or watch the things you gave your life to, broken,
And stoop and build 'em up with worn-out tools;

If you can make one heap of all your winnings
And risk it on one turn of pitch-and-toss,
And lose, and start again at your beginnings
And never breathe a word about your loss;
If you can force your heart and nerve and sinew
To serve your turn long after they are gone,
And so hold on when there is nothing in you
Except the Will which says to them: "Hold on!"

If you can talk with crowds and keep your virtue,
Or walk with Kings — nor lose the common touch,
If neither foes nor loving friends can hurt you,

Dr. Johnny E. Brown

If all men count with you, but none too much;
If you can fill the unforgiving minute
With sixty seconds' worth of distance run --
Yours is the Earth and everything that's in it,
And -- which is more -- you'll be a Man, my son!

Part Four

Reading Words Definitions (Abbreviated)

1. Absolution — Act of forgiving someone for having done something wrong.
2. Amalgamation — The action or process of uniting or merging of two or more things. To merge into a single body.
3. Ambivalence — Simultaneous and contradictory attitudes and feelings toward an object, person, or action.
4. Antebellum — Existing before a war, especially before the American Civil War.
5. Assiduously — Showing great care, attention, and effort; marked by careful . . . attention or persistent application.
6. Avarice — Excessive or insatiable desire for wealth or gain: greediness.
7. Beguiling — Agreeably or charmingly attractive or pleasing. Crafty. Cunning. Artful.

8. Benighted - To be . . . overtaken by darkness or night. Existing in a state of intellectual, moral, or social darkness. Uneducated.

9. Buoyant - Cheerful, gay, capable of maintaining a satisfactorily high level.

10. Capacious - Containing or capable of containing a great deal . . . roomy, spacious.

11. Cataclysm - Flood. Deluge. Catastrophe. Momentous and violent event marked by overwhelming upheaval and demolition.

12. Clamorous - Marked by confused din or outcry . . . noisily insistent. Loud. Emotional.

13. Conviviality - Relating to, occupied with, or fond of feasting, drinking, and good company.

14. Decadence - A period of decay or decline or falling from a higher to a lower level in quality, character of vitality.

15. Disconsolate - Cheerless. Dejected, downcast.

16. Egalitarianism - A belief in human equality especially with respect to social, political, and economic affairs. Social philosophy advocating the removal of inequalities among people.

17. Enmity - Active and typically mutual hatred or ill will. Hostility. Antagonism. Animosity.

18. Expostulated - Discussed, examined. To reason earnestly with a person for purposes of dissuasion.

19. Fictive - Not genuine. Of or relating to, or capable of imaginative creation. Fictional.

20. Homiletic - The art of preaching. Related to a sermon, lecture on a moral theme, moralistic.

21. Implacable - Not capable of being appeased, significantly changed, or mitigated. Adamant.

22. Impudence - Marked by contemptuous or cocky boldness or disregard of others. Insolent. Lacking modesty.

23. Impunity - Exemption or freedom from punishment, harm, or loss.

24. Indefatigable - Incapable of being fatigued. Untiring. Tireless.
25. Ineffaceably - Ineradicable – unable to be eradicated . . . Unable to be erased or forgotten.
26. Intelligible - Capable of being understood or comprehended.
27. Intemperance - Lack of moderation. Especially – habitual or excessive drinking or intoxicants.
28. Loquacity - The quality of being very talkative.
29. Magnanimity - Showing or suggesting a lofty and courageous spirit. Showing or suggesting nobility of feeling and generosity of mind.
30. Mellifluous - Having a smooth, rich flow. Mellow. Melodious. Musical.
31. Mendacity - Given to or characterized by deception or falsehood or divergence from absolute truth.
32. Non-Sequitur - An inference that does not follow from the premises. A statement (such as response) that does not follow logically from or is not clearly related to anything previously said.
33. Ostentatious - Attracting or seeking to attract attention, admiration, or envy often by gaudiness or obviousness. Overly elaborate or conspicuous. Flamboyant. Flashy. Loud. Noisy.
34. Pacifism - Opposition to war or violence as a means of settling disputes. Refusal to bear arms on moral or religious grounds. An attitude or policy of nonresistance.
35. Peripatetic - Pedestrian. Itinerant. Movement or journeys hither and thither. Moving or traveling from place to place.
36. Poignant - Painfully affecting the feelings. Designed to make an impression. Pleasurably stimulating. Impactful. Impressive. Moving.
37. Polemical - Controversial. An aggressive attack on or refutation of the opinions or principles of another.

38. Precociousness - Exceptionally early in development or occurrence. Exhibiting mature qualities at an unusually early age.

39. Profligate - Wildly extravagant in spending. A person given to wildly extravagant and usually grossly self-indulgent expenditure.

40. Prolific - Producing young or fruit especially freely. Fruitful. Causing abundant growth, generation, or reproduction. Marked by abundant inventiveness or productivity.

41. Propitious - Favorably disposed. Benevolent. Auspicious. Tending to favor. Advantageous. Encouraging. Hopeful.

42. Rapacity - Greedy. Gluttonous. Living on prey. Excessively grasping or covetous.

43. Rebuked - To criticize sharply. Reprimand. To turn back or keep down. Expression of strong disapproval.

44. Regal - Of notable excellence or magnificence. Splendid. Kingly. Queenly. Royal.

45. Repartee - A quick and witty reply. A succession or interchange of clever retorts. Amusing and usually light sparring with words.

46. Reproach - An expression of rebuke or disapproval. The act or action of . . . disapproving. A cause or occasion of blame, discredit, or disgrace.

47. Revelatory - Serving to reveal something. Revealing. Suggestive.

48. Salacious - Arousing or appealing to sexual desire or imagination. Lecherous. Lustful.

49. Stultifying - To have a dulling or inhibiting effect on. To impair. Invalidate, or make ineffective. Negate. To cause to appear or be stupid, foolish, or absurdly illogical.

50. Stupendous   - Causing astonishment or wonder. Awesome. Marvelous. Of amazing size or greatness. Tremendous.
51. Suasion   - The act of influencing or persuading.
52. Tempestuous   - Turbulent. Stormy. Fierce. Furious.
53. Ubiquitous   - Existing or being everywhere at the same time.
54. Virulently   - A . . . virulent infection marked by rapid, severe, and destructive force. Able to overcome bodily defensive mechanisms. Extremely poisonous or venomous.

References

Blight, D. W. (2018). *Frederick Douglass: Prophet of freedom*. New York, NY: Simon & Schuster.

Brown, J. (2020). *The Emerson Street story: Race, class, quality of life and faith*. Bloomington, IN: AuthorHOUSE.

Henley, W. (1875). Invictus. In R. Cook (Ed.), (1997). In *101 famous poems*. New York, NY: McGraw-Hill.

Johnson, J. W. (2006). Lift ev'ry voice and sing (1917). In *The Oxford anthology of African American poetry*. Rampersad, A. (Ed.). New York, NY: Oxford University Press.

The King James Version Study Bible. Edward E. Hindson (Ed.). (2017). Liberty University. HarperCollins Christian Publishing.

Kipling, R. (1895). If. In *ID voice: vision: identity*. (pp.88-89). New York, NY: Scholastic, Inc.

Merriam-Webster's collegiate dictionary (2021). Springfield, MA: Merriam-Webster, Inc.

Publications/Papers

- Brown, J. (1991). <u>Leader behavior and school effectiveness.</u> Ann Arbor: University Microfilms International (U.M.I.). Dissertation – <u>Leader behavior and school effectiveness.</u> Focus on a) site management and b) principals' leadership relative to instruction and home-school relations.

- Encyclopedia Article: Akins, W., & Brown, J. (1993). Sweatt v. Painter (1950) In Anderson, D., Asbury, C., Jones-Wilson, F., & Okazawa-Rey (Eds.). <u>The Encyclopedia of African American Education</u>.

- Brown, J. (1991). <u>Leader behavior and school effectiveness</u>. Paper presented at the annual meeting of the American Educational Research Association in Chicago, Illinois. Unpublished paper based upon research findings.

- Brown, J. (2020). The Emerson Street Story: Race, Class, Quality of Life and Faith. Bloomington, IN. AuthorHouse.

Web site: www.jcbil.com
Twitter: @jbrowneducator
www.facebook.com/johnny.e.brown.7/

Logo for Johnny & Carolyn Brown Institute for Learning

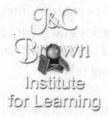

LOGO FOR WAPP – Author & Mary
(Brown) Ruegg

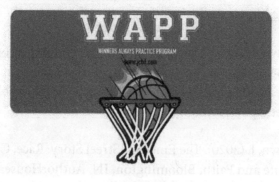

About the Author

Dr. Johnny Edward Brown is a native of Austin, Texas, residing during his early life on Emerson Street. He graduated from the original L. C. Anderson High School, where he was a member of the varsity basketball team. He became the first African American athlete for an intercollegiate athletic program at Southwest Texas State University (Texas State University) in San Marcos, Texas. Dr. Brown worked as a teacher-coach early in his career, first at the middle school level in San Antonio and then Austin, where he became the first high school varsity head basketball coach at the current L. C. Anderson High School. Dr. Brown has served as an administrative leader, including principal and superintendent, for schools and school districts in four states. He earned the Bachelor of Science in Education and Master of Education degrees at Texas State University, and the terminal degree, Doctor of Philosophy, at the University of Texas at Austin. He has completed post-graduate work and serves as an adjunct professor at Lamar University in Beaumont, Texas. He routinely speaks to various audiences regarding the successful education of our youth. Dr. Brown is an active volunteer in his community. He and his wife, Carolyn, also an educator, are members of the St. Peter's United Methodist Church in Austin and regular attendees and supporters of the Antioch Missionary Baptist Church of Beaumont. They are parents of a son, two daughters, two sons-in-law, and one granddaughter. Dr. Brown is the author of the book: The Emerson Street Story: Race, Class, Quality of Life and Faith (2020).